I0414416

The HAPI Heart Diet

The HAPI Heart Diet

A COMMON-SENSE APPROACH TO
A HAPPY AND HEART-HEALTHY LIFE

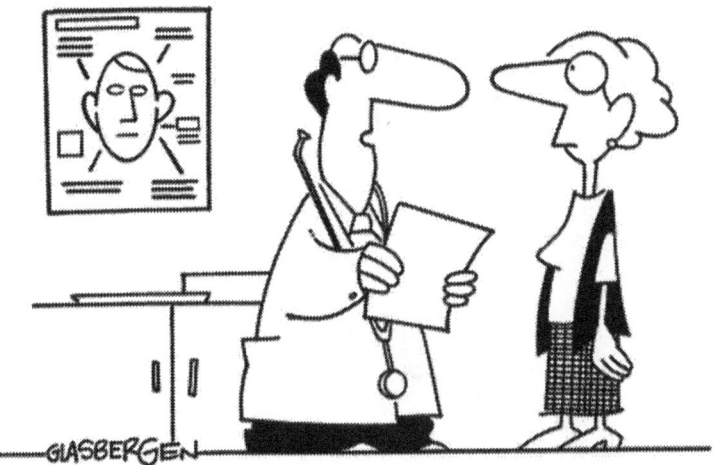

© 1999 Randy Glasbergen. www.glasbergen.com

GLASBERGEN

"You've got a rare condition called 'good health'.
Frankly, we're not sure how to treat it."

Dr. Michael P. Varveris, M.D.

Medical Director, Heart Attack Prevention Institute (HAPI), Naples, Florida

iUniverse, Inc.
New York Lincoln Shanghai

The HAPI Heart Diet
A Common-Sense Approach to a Happy and Heart-Healthy Life

Copyright © 2006 by Michael P. Varveris

All rights reserved. No part of this book may be used or reproduced by any means, graphic, electronic, or mechanical, including photocopying, recording, taping or by any information storage retrieval system without the written permission of the publisher except in the case of brief quotations embodied in critical articles and reviews.

iUniverse books may be ordered through booksellers or by contacting:

iUniverse
2021 Pine Lake Road, Suite 100
Lincoln, NE 68512
www.iuniverse.com
1-800-Authors (1-800-288-4677)

This book is intended for informational purposes only.
It contains a mixture of generally accepted medical facts as well as personal medical opinions. In no way does it serve as a replacement for seeing a physician for medical care and individual medical decision-making or a dietician/nutritionist or exercise physiologist for personalized dietary/lifestyle/exercise recommendations.

ISBN-13: 978-0-595-38895-0 (pbk)
ISBN-13: 978-0-595-84856-0 (cloth)
ISBN-13: 978-0-595-83273-6 (ebk)
ISBN-10: 0-595-38895-7 (pbk)
ISBN-10: 0-595-84856-7 (cloth)
ISBN-10: 0-595-83273-3 (ebk)

Printed in the United States of America

Contents

Copyright 2002 by Randy Glasbergen.   www.glasbergen.com

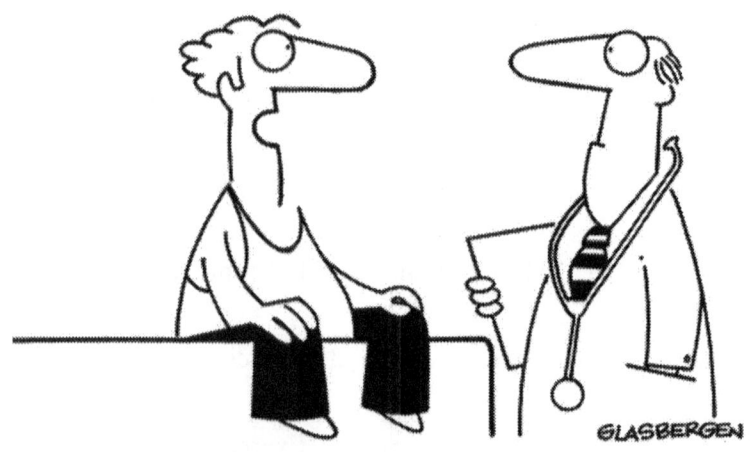

"Eat less and exercise more? That's the
most ridiculous fad diet I've heard of yet!"

Acknowledgments

To my mother, Kanella Stanos Varveris, for being willing to sacrifice anything to help me become a physician

To my father, Michael Nicholas Varveris, for serving as my role model in writing and publishing a book

To my multi-talented wife, Nicola, and beautiful daughters, Ariana Eleni and Alexandra Persephone, for being the loves of my life

To Drs. Paul Ziajka, William Cromwell and Bradley Bale, for exposing me to the connection between lipoproteins, type 2 diabetes mellitus and atherosclerotic cardiovascular disease and Drs. Arthur Agatston, Douglas Brewer and John Rumberger, for inspiring me to follow in their footsteps and write a diet/lifestyle book from a physician's perspective

To my good friend, Bobby Watson, for recognizing and nurturing my passion for sharing my scientific beliefs with my peers in clinical medicine

To Dr. Thomas Dayspring, for continuing education on lipoprotein physiology/pathology as well as sharing some mighty cool graphics

To my good friend, Professor James Price, for the wonderful culinary photography

To Mr. Randy Glasbergen (www.glasbergen.com), for all the clever diet-, exercise-and cholesterol-related cartoons

Copyright 2002 by Randy Glasbergen.
www.glasbergen.com

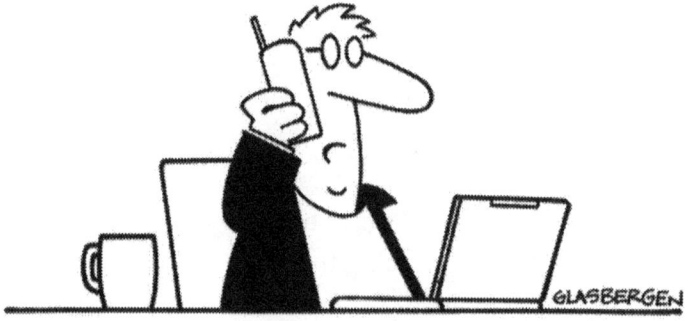

"I'd like to order a gift basket filled with chocolates, sausages, cheesecake, a bottle of whiskey and a carton of cigarettes. It's for my doctor."

Why I Wrote 'Another' Diet Book

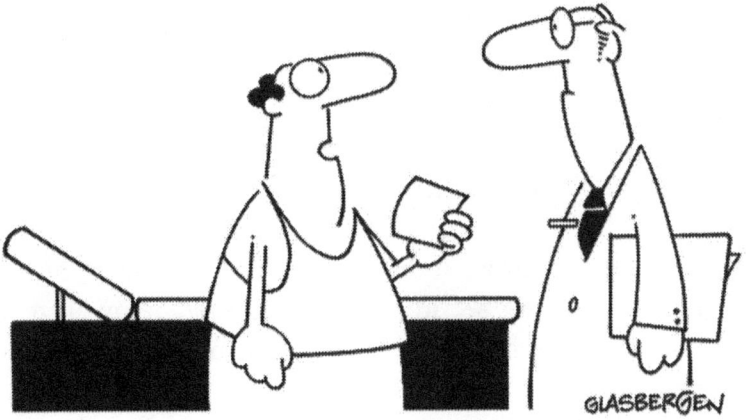

Copyright 2005 by Randy Glasbergen.
www.glasbergen.com

GLASBERGEN

"Which 'sensible diet' do you want me to follow?
I found 123,942 of them on the internet!"

Q: How much training in diet, exercise and nutrition does the typical physician have in medical school and/or in internship/residency/fellowship following medical school?

A. None

Patients come to doctors for solutions to their problems. One of the biggest (no pun intended) problems occurring in our modern society is obesity and the associated disease states of type 2 diabetes mellitus and atherosclerotic cardiovascular disease. In such circumstances, the physician will typically advise the patient to: "Exercise and follow a sensible diet." But the conversation usually ends at that point. This book is my attempt to continue the discussion.

I have always believed the most important questions to have answered are of the 'How' and 'Why' type. Therefore, in this book, we will first discuss how and why lipoprotein ('cholesterol') disorders serve as the linchpin for obesity, type 2 diabetes as well as cardiovascular disease. These concepts will be discussed in some detail—hopefully for the interest and education of patients as well as physicians.

Since the 'truth' usually resides between the two extremes of 'ignorance' and 'neurosis,' we will then elucidate on various nutritional-, dietary-and exercise-related concepts to find some common sense recommendations for happy and heart-healthy living. The five central principles of the HAPI Heart Diet will be described: 1) eating less; 2) eating smarter; 3) exercising more; 4) exercising smarter; and 5) having the right attitude. This section will also include many of my favorite delicious, yet health-conscious recipes. Following this will be a chapter intended for physicians (as well as any other interested parties) regarding recent important medical advances in the diagnosis and treatment of lipoprotein disorders.

Regardless of whether or not other diets have worked for you in the past, if you think positively ('have the right attitude'), decrease your daily caloric intake ('eat less'), increase your daily caloric expenditure ('exercise more'), optimize your daily metabolism ('eat smarter' and 'exercise smarter') and realize you are embracing a new and better way of life rather than a new and better way to fit into some trendy clothes for your upcoming high school reunion, you will find it impossible not to succeed with this approach.

The HAPI Heart Diet isn't for the guy who's just come from the doctor's office, a little shell-shocked at having received the news that his total cholesterol is in the 250+ range nor for the health-conscious couple that simply wants to acquire a new repertoire of recipes and restock their fridge. This book is for people who are serious about understanding cardiovascular disease as well as changing their lives for the better. This book is not light and fluffy, like so many other diet, exercise and 'healthy living' books. The HAPI Heart Diet isn't for weenies. This isn't a 'dance your way to better health, pour a glass of wine and let's talk about cutting out butter' book. No gimmick, no quick fix and no miracle pill will be found in these pages.

The underlying theme of the HAPI Heart Diet is more like: 'I'm talking to you as an adult responsible for your own health; I will not sugar coat what I believe to be the truth; I will not talk down to you; I will not make it easy but I <u>WILL</u> keep it as simple and straight-forward as possible.' Please be appreciative, rather than alarmed or offended, by my level of frankness. Readers will have to roll up their sleeves and pay attention, but they will learn everything they need to know about lipoprotein subclasses, physiologic versus pathologic conditions, 'good' versus 'bad' fats and will walk away with all kinds of diet and exercise advice, eclectic health-and nutrition-related tips and even some yummy recipes.

I have included specialized information (including an entire additional chapter) meant primarily for physicians because I want the doctor and patient to be on equal footing and the 'same page' when it comes to health, disease, exercise and proper nutrition. Be prepared for statistics, graphs and in-depth medical terminology to be presented from the outset. Don't worry—you <u>WILL</u> understand the 'big picture' nature of any technical scientific lingo. I throw a wide net in the HAPI Heart Diet and hope to ensnare you, reel you in and share with you (whether prospective patient or clinician) a thing or two about happy, heart-healthy living.

In my opinion, life is a blessing and gift from the Creator whose purpose is the continuous improvement of our self and of others around us. We are challenged with many choices throughout our life in this journey of self-improvement. It is the choices we make that help determine our future. We are motivated in these choices either by love or by fear. This book is my attempt to help patients and doctors make better choices for healthier and happier futures based on love for life rather than fear of sickness or death. My intent was to present my thoughts for the reader's education, inspiration and enjoyment. I truly hope this book makes a positive impact upon your life.

Michael P. Varveris, MD ('Dr. V')
12/26/05

♘

Chapter One
Lipoproteins, Cardiovascular Disease, Metabolic Syndrome and Type 2 Diabetes

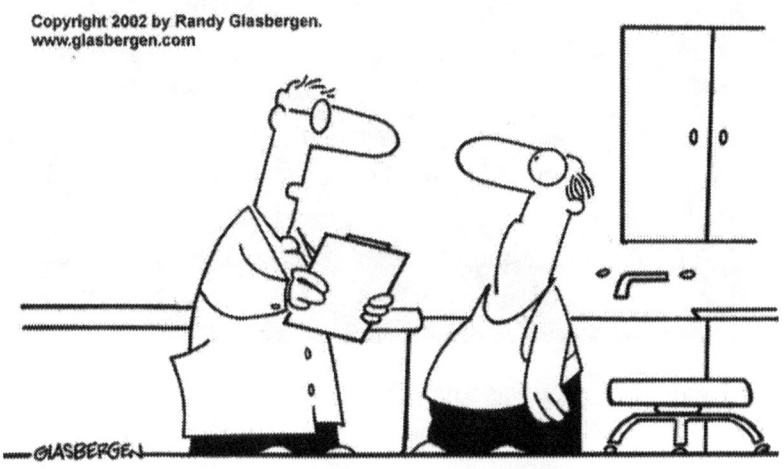

Copyright 2002 by Randy Glasbergen.
www.glasbergen.com

GLASBERGEN

"No, HDL and LDL were not the robots in Star Wars."

Cardiovascular (CV) disease is becoming a global pandemic (see Image 1 below), pretty much the number one cause of premature death (heart attack, sudden cardiac death) and definitely the number one cause of premature permanent disability (stroke) in the United States and rest of the industrialized world. To put things into perspective, more Americans die every single day from CV disease than all the people murdered by radical Islamo-fascist terrorists on 9/11/01 (see Image 2 below). Despite medical advances in the recognition and management of CV disease, the likelihood of CV events during the lifetime of the typical 'healthy' (non-smoking, non-obese, non-hypertensive, non-diabetic) 40-year old adult remains very high—almost 49% for men and 32% for women (see Image 3 below).

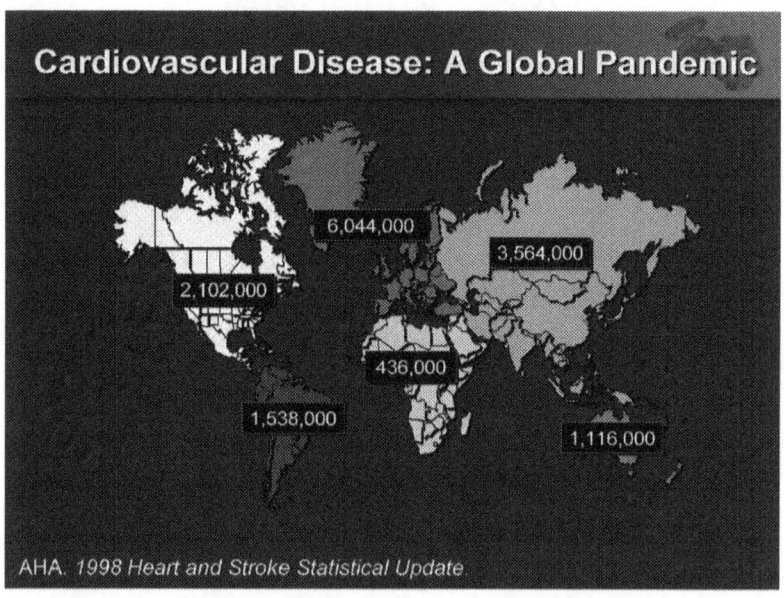

Image 1: Cardiovascular Disease: A Global Pandemic

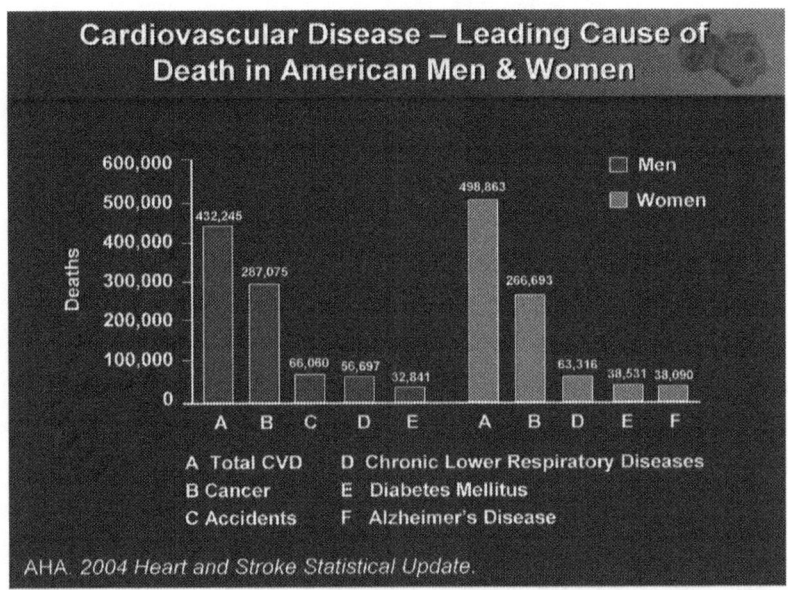

Image 2: Cardiovascular Disease—Leading Cause of Death in American Men & Women

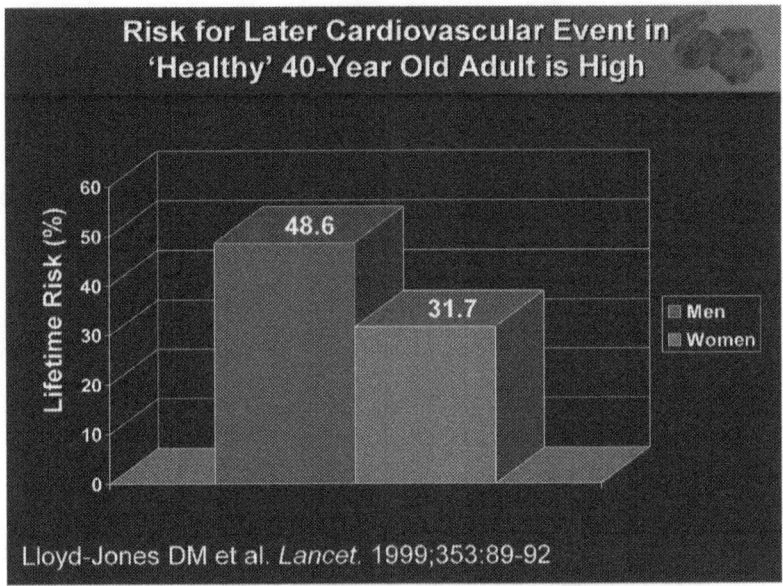

Image 3: Risk for Later Cardiovascular Event in 'Healthy' 40-Year Old Adult is High

When we manage (as patients and doctors) CV disease, we focus on managing the risk factors for this condition (see Image 4 below). These risk factors include those that are non-modifiable (genetics, gender, ethnicity, the aging process) as well as those that are completely modifiable (lifestyle choices, hypertension, diabetes and 'cholesterol' problems—the latter termed dyslipoproteinemia). There is obviously strong interaction between the non-modifiable and modifiable risk factors. If the non-modifiable risk factors 'load the gun' in terms of future CV risk, it's the modifiable ones that 'pull the trigger.' Therefore, we focus on the modifiable risk factors, since they're the ones we're able to influence and alter. All the modifiable risk factors are important but, since CV disease develops and progresses due to inappropriate deposition of cholesterol within the walls of our arterial system (see Image 5 below—the best non-invasive way to identify this process is the carotid intima-media thickness [CIMT] test by CardioRisk [www.cardiorisk.us]), dyslipoproteinemia (abnormalities of lipoprotein particles that transport cholesterol and triglyceride in our bloodstream) is probably the most influential of all the modifiable risk factors.

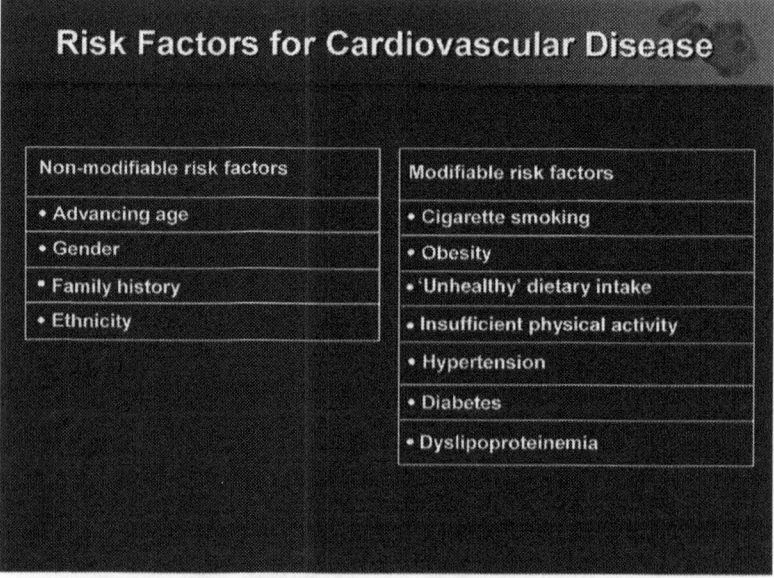

Risk Factors for Cardiovascular Disease

Non-modifiable risk factors	Modifiable risk factors
• Advancing age	• Cigarette smoking
• Gender	• Obesity
• Family history	• 'Unhealthy' dietary intake
• Ethnicity	• Insufficient physical activity
	• Hypertension
	• Diabetes
	• Dyslipoproteinemia

Image 4. Risk Factors for Cardiovascular Disease

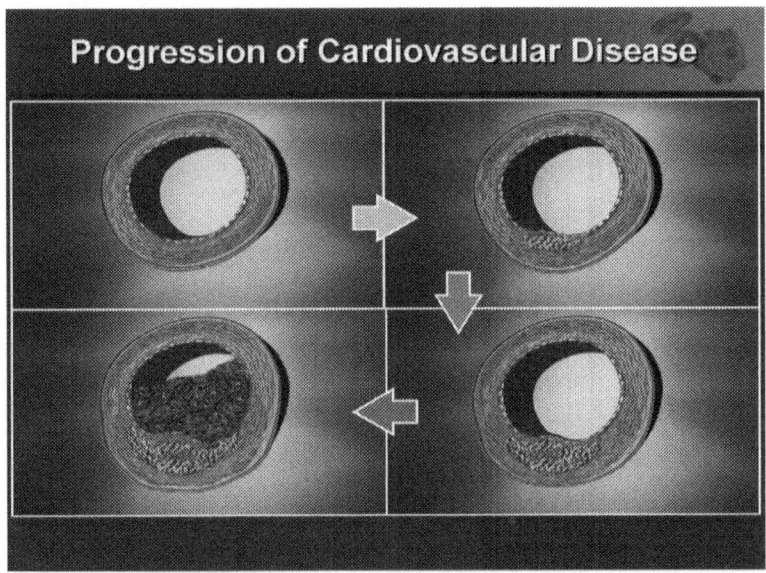

Image 5. Progression of Cardiovascular Disease

The lipoproteins that exist within the bloodstream can be differentiated from one another by their size as well as by their density (see Image 6 below). Lipoproteins (lipo [fat] + protein) are just what the name implies, spherical particles with fats (cholesterol and triglyceride) in their cores and proteins embedded into their surfaces (see Image 7 below). These surface proteins allow lipoprotein particles to interact with various receptors, proteins and enzymes within our body. The more fat relative to protein these particles contain, the more buoyant they are while the less fat relative to protein they contain, the more dense they are. Imagine a glass of water (the bloodstream is an aqueous medium). If you pour some olive oil (fat) into that glass, the oil will float on the surface (buoyant) while if you drop a piece of meat (protein) into that glass, the meat will sink to the bottom (dense). Think of laboratory measurements of lipids (total cholesterol [TC], LDL-cholesterol [LDL-C], HDL-cholesterol [HDL-C] and triglyceride [TG]) as 'shadow markers' of the actual lipoprotein particle concentrations.

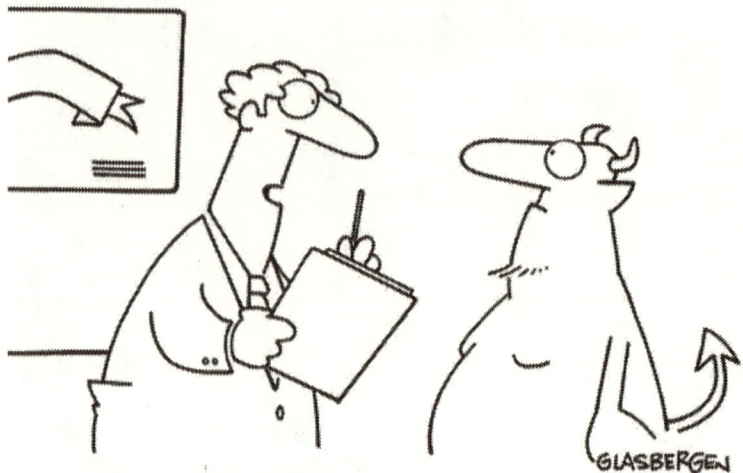

Copyright 2005 by Randy Glasbergen. www.glasbergen.com

"I know how to treat good cholesterol and bad cholesterol, but this is my first experience with evil cholesterol."

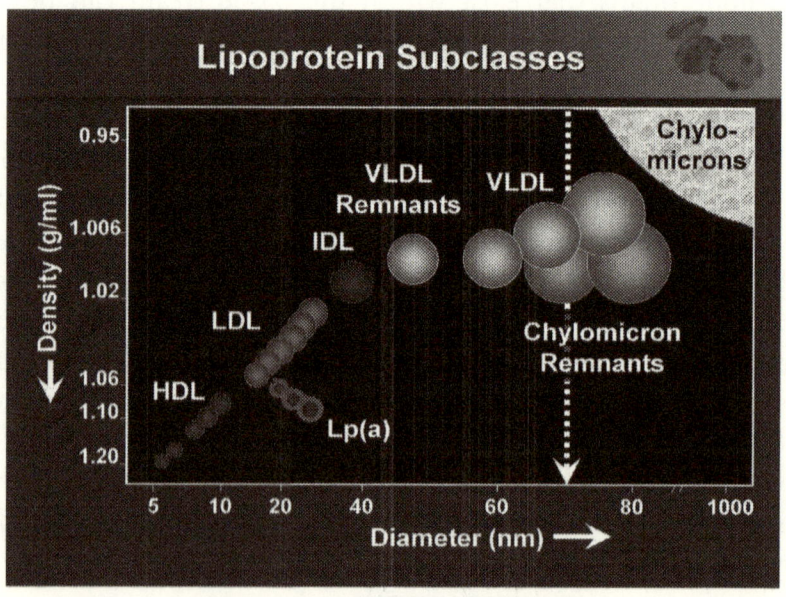

Image 6. Lipoprotein Subclasses

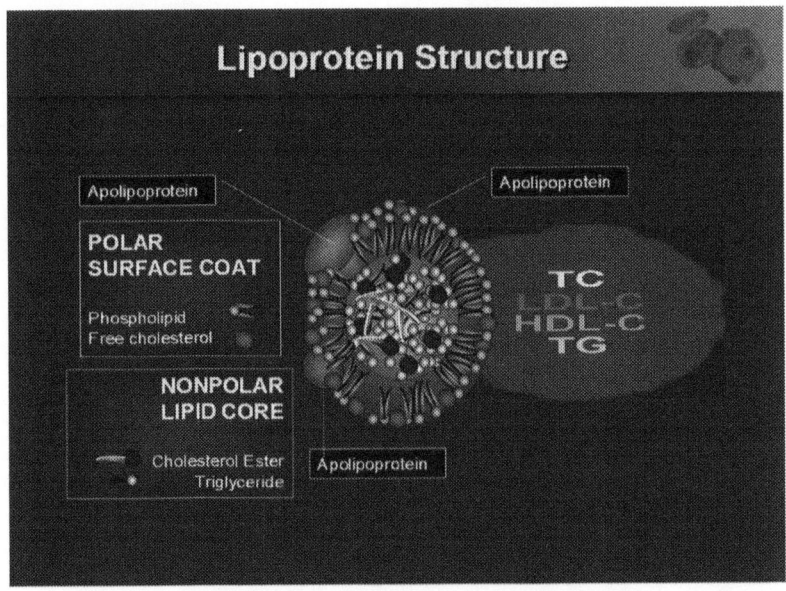

Image 7. Lipoprotein Structure

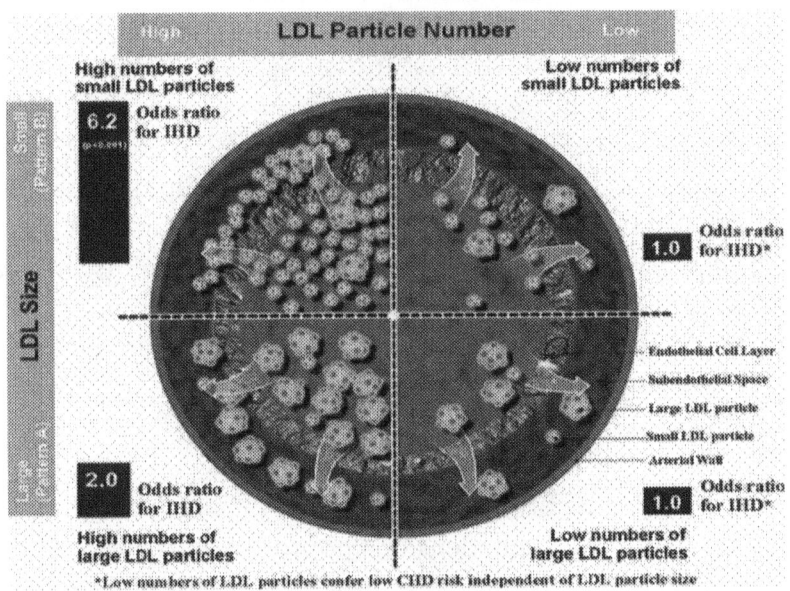

Image 8. Cardiovascular Risk Depends on LDL Particle Number and LDL Particle Size

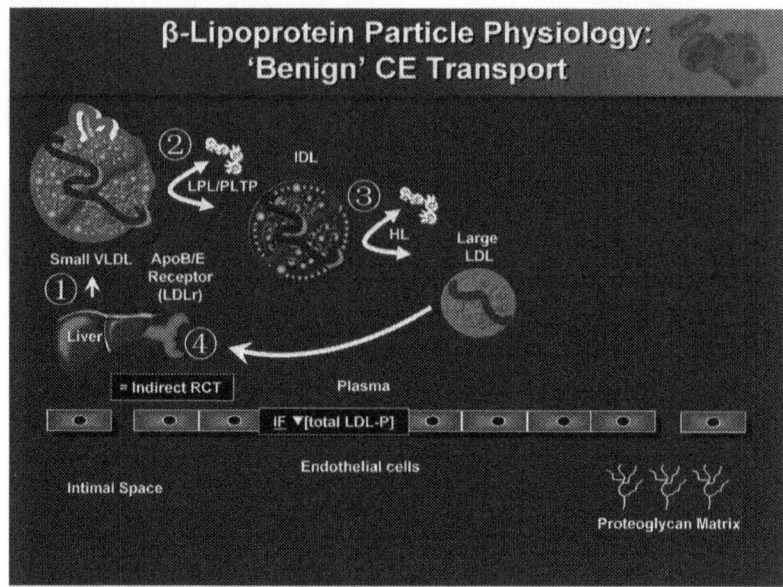

Image 9. β-Lipoprotein Particle Physiology:
'Benign' CE Transport

What can shadows really tell us? If there was a shadow of a man and another shadow of a horse on a wall, even a three-year old child could distinguish the sources of those shadows. What about detail? What color are the man's eyes? Shadows can't tell you detail—lipids can't give you detailed information about lipoproteins. And many times this detail is required to make important clinical decisions. How tall is the man? If his shadow measures 5'9", he could actually be 5' tall or maybe even 6'6" tall—right? Shadows can significantly over-or underestimate the size of things—lipids can significantly over-or underestimate the actual number of lipoprotein particles that exist.

Lipoproteins can be broken down into various subclasses: alpha(α)-lipoproteins (HDL or high density lipoprotein particles); as well as beta(β)-lipoproteins (chylomicron particles and chylomicron remnant [CM-R] particles made by the gut and VLDL or very low density lipoprotein particles, IDL or intermediate density lipoprotein particles and LDL or low density lipoprotein particles produced by the liver). HDL particles are 'good' since, when in excess, they may lead to cholesterol removal from arterial walls while β-lipoproteins (those smaller than 70 nm in diameter) are 'bad' since, when in excess, they may lead to cholesterol deposition within arterial walls.

When cholesterol deposition exists within arterial walls, it is almost always due to excess β-lipoproteins rather than diminished α-lipoproteins. Imagine a bucket (representing the arterial wall) with β-lipoproteins being a measuring cup adding water (cholesterol) to the bucket and α-lipoproteins being a separate measuring cup removing water from the bucket. In the physiologic state, both measuring cups are basically the same size. In the pathologic state, the measuring cup adding water is larger than that removing water so the bucket fills. Thus, when cholesterol deposition exists within arterial walls, the focus is on reducing the concentrations of β-lipoproteins (if the measuring cup adding water is made smaller than that removing water, eventually the bucket will empty).

The most likely β-lipoprotein to deposit cholesterol within arterial walls is the LDL particle. LDL particles come in different sizes—small as well as large. LDL-C usually represents large LDL particles while HDL-C and TG usually represent small LDL particles. Small LDL particles seem more likely to deposit cholesterol within arterial walls than large LDL particles. When the number of total LDL particles in the bloodstream is low, the likelihood that any one of those particles will penetrate arterial walls and deposit cholesterol is low and thus the future CV risk is low. However, when the number of total LDL particles is elevated, there is an increased likelihood that some of those particles will penetrate arterial walls and deposit cholesterol and therefore the future CV risk is elevated (double normal risk if the LDL particles are large but 620% greater than normal risk if the LDL particles are small—see Image 8 above).

Under physiologic conditions (individuals who exercise daily, don't overeat and maintain an appropriate body weight), the liver produces a relatively low number of small VLDL particles (see Image 9 above). 1) These small VLDL particles are secreted by the liver into the bloodstream.

2) They are first converted into IDL particles. 3) The resultant IDL particles are then converted into large LDL particles. 4) The relatively low number of large LDL particles can be recognized by certain receptors on liver cells and removed from the bloodstream to complete a 'benign' cholesterol circuit. It is termed benign since the low numbers of large LDL particles are unlikely to deposit cholesterol within arterial walls.

© 1997 by Randy Glasbergen.

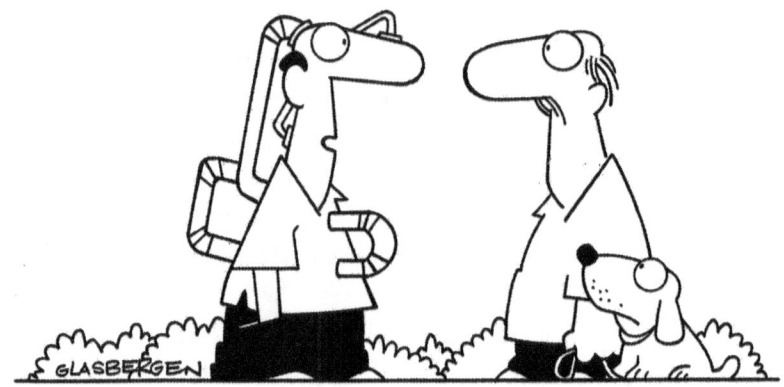

"I installed all new plumbing. I got tired
of fretting about my cholesterol!"

Under pathologic conditions (individuals who overeat, don't exercise and are overweight), the liver produces a relatively increased number of large VLDL particles (see Image 10 below). 1) These large VLDL particles have much more triglyceride in their cores than normal. 2) The large VLDL particles can interact with large LDL particles to convert the latter into small LDL particles. 3) The large VLDL particles are also themselves converted into small LDL particles. 4) As mentioned above, these small LDL particles seem very likely (if in increased number) to penetrate and become entrapped within arterial walls. 5) The small LDL particles are very poorly recognized by hepatic receptors. 6) The entrapped small LDL particles are modified by an oxidative process (the best marker for this being elevated blood levels of lipoprotein-associated phospholipase

A$_2$ [Lp-PLA$_2$—www.diadexus.com]). 7) This oxidative modification leads to the synthesis and release of various inflammatory substances into the bloodstream. 8) Lp-PLA$_2$ can (theoretically) itself lead to small LDL particles. 9) Certain white blood cells (called monocytes) are attracted to the localized inflammation, penetrate the arterial wall, are converted into activated macrophages and engulf the modified small LDL particles to complete a 'malignant' cholesterol circuit. It is termed malignant since the activated macrophages (induced by high numbers of entrapped small LDL particles) lead to cholesterol build-up within arterial walls and eventually CV disease.

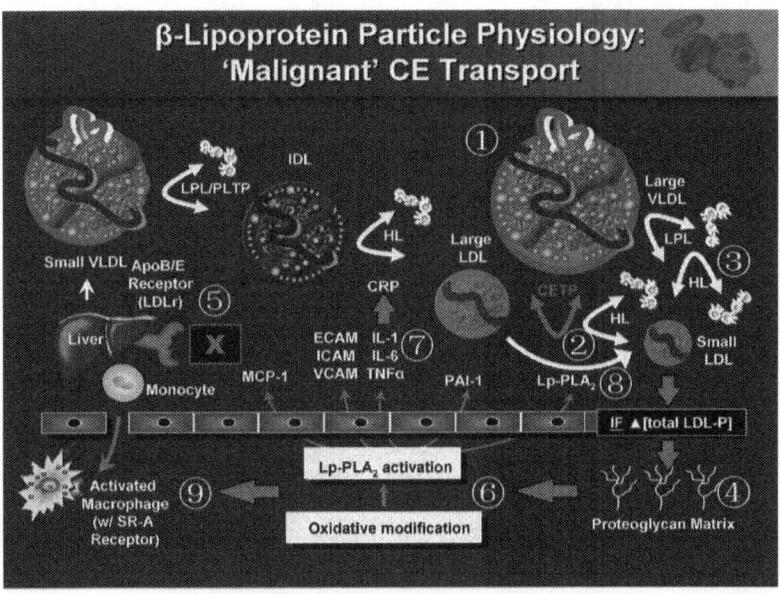

Image 10. β-Lipoprotein Particle Physiology: 'Malignant' CE Transport

When the concentration of 'fat' (cholesterol and/or triglyceride) within the liver is increased (due to genetic as well as lifestyle factors), the liver responds by increasing its production of β-lipoproteins as well as decreasing its removal of β-lipoproteins from the bloodstream. If that fat is primarily cholesterol (from genetics more so than lifestyle), the resultant increased β-lipoproteins are mainly large LDL particles. On the other hand, if the fat is primarily triglyceride (from lifestyle more so than genetics), the resultant increased β-lipoproteins are mainly small LDL particles.

Another important modifiable risk factor to consider is 'metabolic syndrome' (MS)—also termed insulin resistance (IR), pre-diabetes and/or syndrome X. This condition occurs because of unwise lifestyle choices—lack of appropriate physical activity, excessive caloric intake and resultant obesity. MS/IR is becoming quite prevalent among American adults, both men as well as women (see Image 11 below). This condition becomes more common the older we get but is actually increasing the most in younger individuals, especially adolescents.

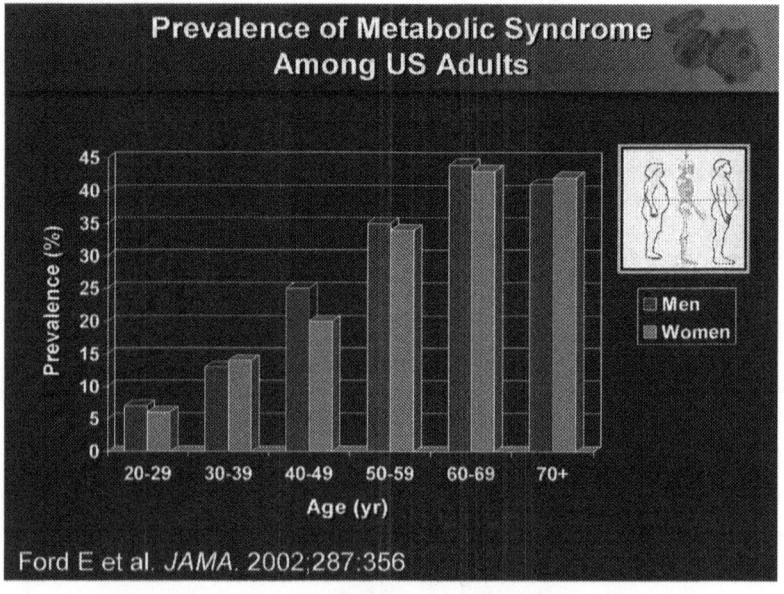

Image 11: Prevalence of Metabolic Syndrome
Among US Adults

The current medical classification of MS/IR includes five clinical parameters: 1) hypertension (HTN); 2) abdominal obesity; 3) elevated serum TG levels; 4) low serum HDL-C levels; and 5) high serum fasting blood glucose (FBG) levels (see Image 12 below). The diagnosis of MS/IR necessitates three or more of these five clinical parameters.

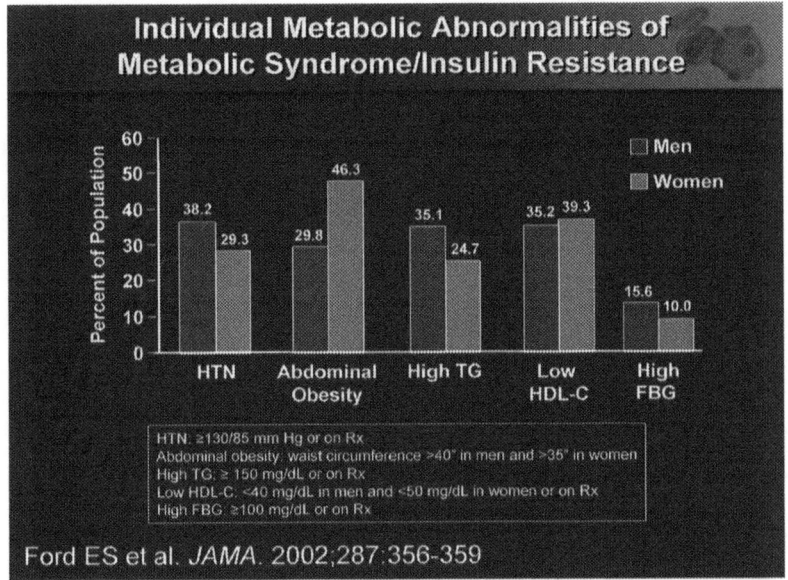

Image 12: Individual Metabolic Abnormalities of
Metabolic Syndrome/Insulin Resistance

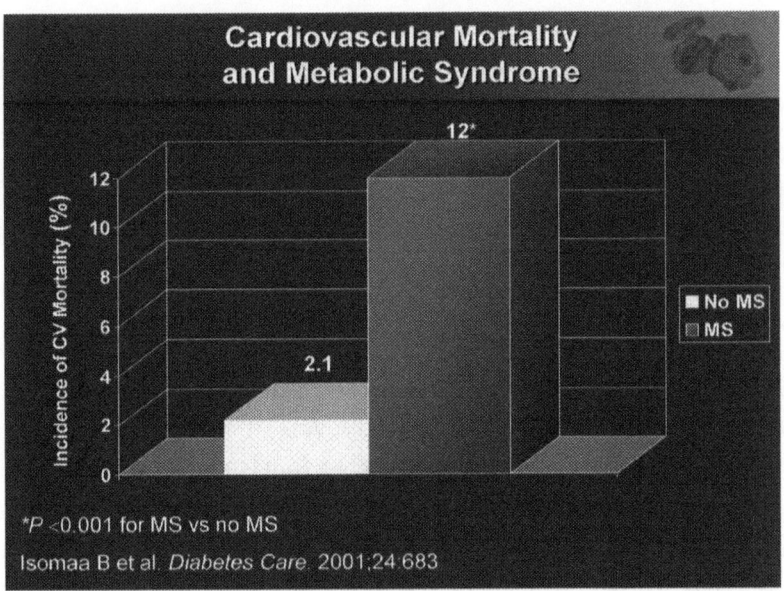

Image 13: Cardiovascular Mortality
and Metabolic Syndrome

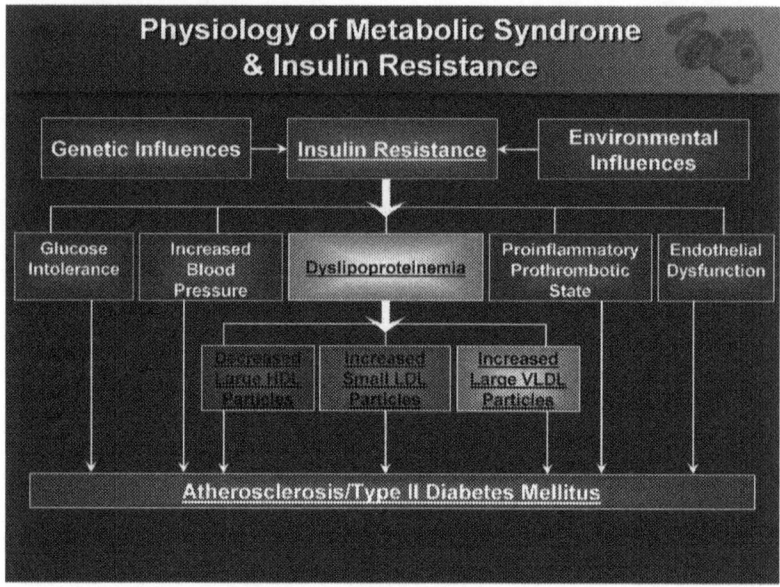

Image 14: Physiology of Metabolic Syndrome
& Insulin Resistance

The presence of MS (compared to its absence) has been shown to increase the likelihood of future CV mortality by up to 600% (see Image 13 above). This increased risk is ENTIRELY reversible, however, if the unwise lifestyle choices that caused the syndrome are corrected. Thus it is IMPERATIVE for anyone having MS/IR to limit their daily caloric consumption as well as increase their daily physical activity level to attain a more appropriate body weight.

If one looks at the actual underlying pathology of MS/IR, one would find that dyslipoproteinemia serves as the linchpin for this disease state (see Image 14 above). Namely, elevated levels of small LDL particles, low levels of large HDL particles and elevated levels of large VLDL particles are the core mechanism of MS/IR. Since in many clinical circumstances, MS/IR actually represents a precursor state to type 2 diabetes mellitus (type II DM), these same three lipoprotein abnormalities also serve as the linchpin for type II DM.

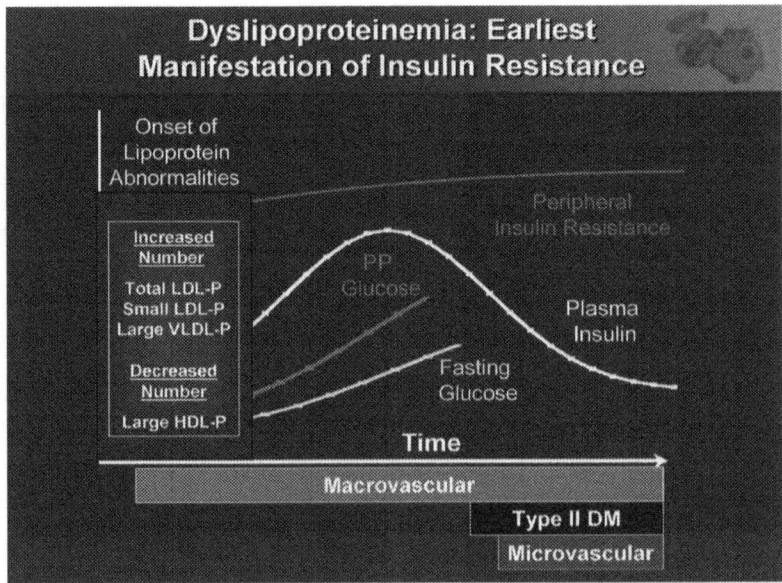

Image 15: Dyslipoproteinemia: Earliest
Manifestation of Insulin Resistance

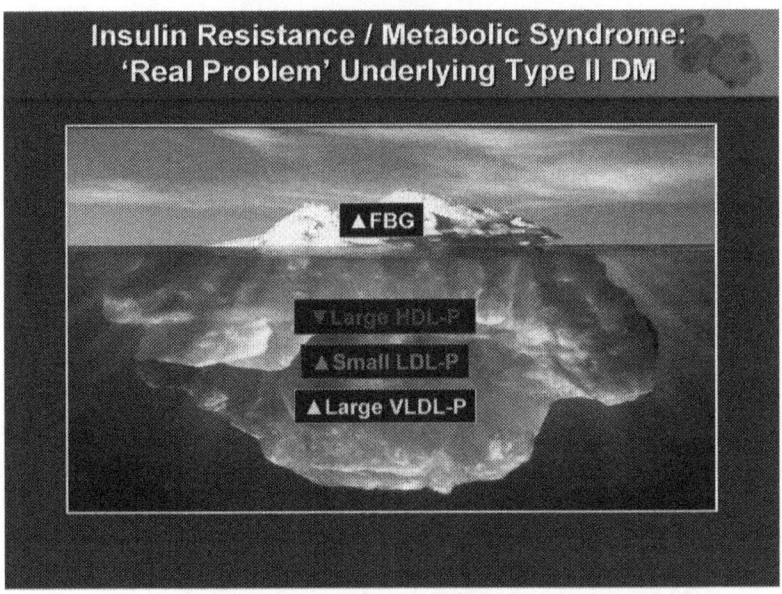

Image 16: Insulin Resistance/Metabolic Syndrome:
'Real Problem' Underlying Type II DM

In fact, abnormal serum lipoprotein concentrations of the type described above can be detected in the bloodstream of those individuals destined to become type 2 diabetics up to 20–25 years before the serum FBG begins to rise (see Image 15 above). Dyslipoproteinemia is the precursor to CV disease in these individuals with heart attacks and/or strokes occurring perhaps years prior to any elevation of FBG and diagnosis of type II DM.

Think of type II DM as an iceberg (see Image 16 above). What sinks your Titanic is not the tip of that iceberg (the elevated FBG) but rather the body of the iceberg that exists beneath the water's surface (the elevated levels of small LDL and large VLDL particles as well as diminished levels of large HDL particles). In fact, the tip of the iceberg basically only serves as a warning that there's a big iceberg lying underneath that you better watch out for—or it <u>WILL</u> sink your Titanic. The best way to rid your body of CV risk from MS/IR as well as type II DM is to eat less, exercise more and lose weight (which will decrease the production of large VLDL as well as small LDL particles and increase the production of large HDL particles). <u>MELT</u> the iceberg and you needn't worry about your Titanic sinking, right?

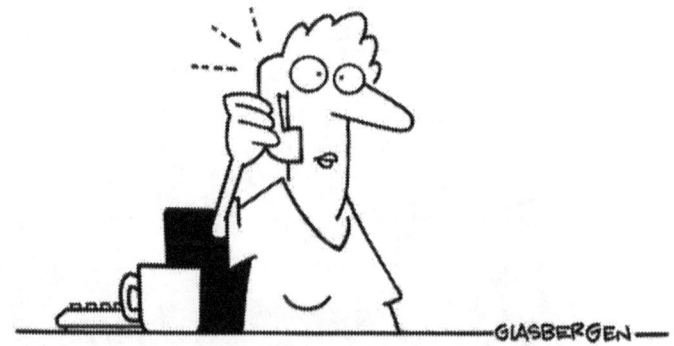

Copyright 2004 by Randy Glasbergen.
www.glasbergen.com

GLASBERGEN

"Welcome to the Diabetic Hotline! If you need a new excuse for cheating on your diet, press 1. If you need a new excuse for skipping your workout, press 2…"

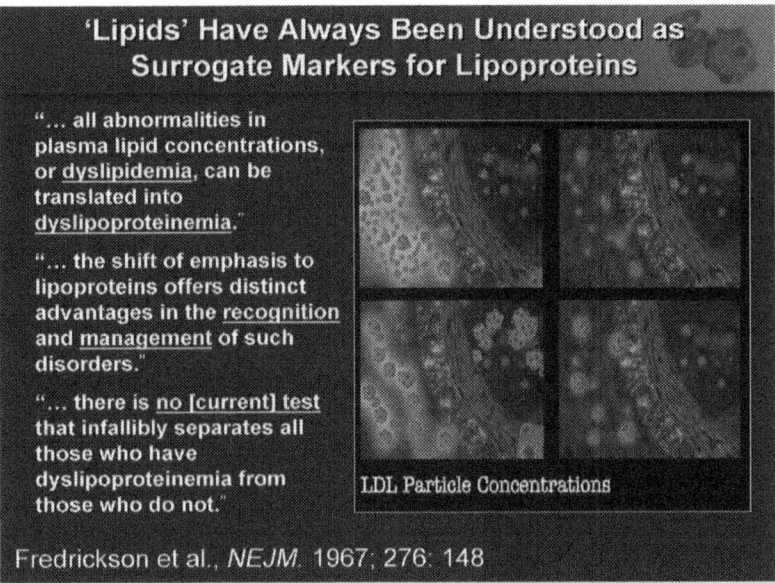

Image 17: Lipids Have Always Been Understood as 'Shadow' Markers for Lipoproteins

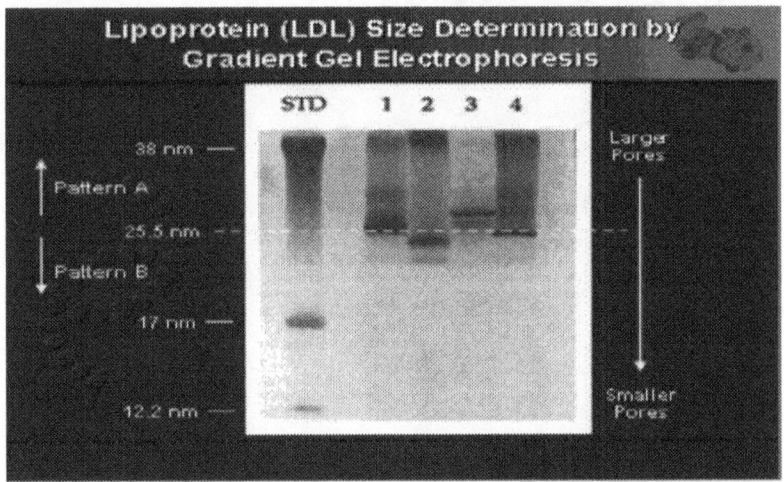

Image 18: Lipoprotein (LDL) Size Determination by Gradient Gel Electrophoresis

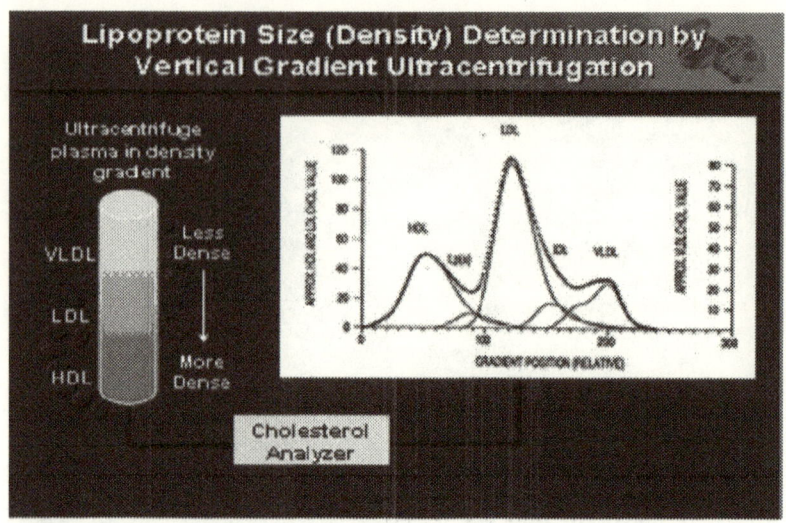

Image 19: Lipoprotein Size (Density) Determination by Vertical Gradient Ultracentrifugation

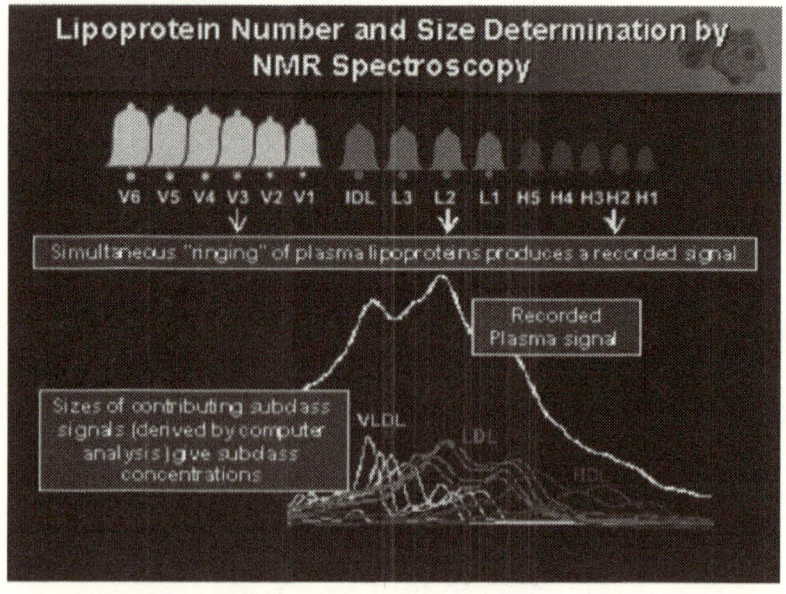

Image 20. Lipoprotein Number and Size Determination by NMR Spectroscopy

So the total number of LDL particles (large and small) determines CV risk and the number of small LDL particles, large VLDL particles and large HDL particles determines the likelihood of becoming a type 2 diabetic. However, what the vast majority of clinicians currently measure are not LDL, HDL and/or VLDL particle numbers but rather surrogate markers of these called LDL-C, HDL-C and TG. These lipid values are nothing but shadows of the actual lipoprotein particle concentrations as discussed above.

The concept that any disorder of serum lipids (dyslipidemia) is just a shadow of the true disease state (dyslipoproteinemia) is not a new one (see Image 17 above). In fact, even in 1967 was it understood that recognizing and managing patients based upon lipoprotein rather than lipid data would obviously be advantageous. But, at that time, it was technically impossible to measure lipoproteins so we have grown accustomed to using lipids as surrogate markers for lipoproteins because 'lipids are better than nothing.' However, three 'advanced' lipid tests have recently become commercially available and finally have provided us the ability to determine large as well as small LDL particle levels (among other such parameters).

The first of these three advanced tests is called segmental gradient gel electrophoresis (SGGE) by Berkeley HeartLab. SGGE separates LDL and HDL particles based upon their size using pores of decreasing diameter embedded into a gel medium through which the lipoproteins migrate. After the lipoproteins have separated, a lipid stain is applied and the relative intensity of stain in each separated LDL and HDL particle subclass is measured (see Image 18 above).

The second test is called vertical auto-profile (VAP) using vertical gradient ultracentrifugation by Atherotech. VAP separates VLDL, LDL and HDL particles based upon their density in a salt solution and then directly measures cholesterol in each separated lipoprotein subclass (see Image 19 above).

The third test is called nuclear magnetic resonance (NMR) spectroscopy by LipoScience [www.liposcience.com]. NMR directly measures lipoprotein particle number in all major lipoprotein subclasses (see Image 20 above) but focuses primarily on total LDL particle number (LDL-P) and small LDL-P. NMR-derived total LDL-P and small LDL-P are the only lipid-related parameters of CV risk that have consistently been shown to remain significant and independent (see Image 21 below) in predicting such risk when modified for other associated clinical parameters (family history, smoking, obesity, blood pressure, FBG, lipids, C-reactive protein [CRP]).

Prospective Outcome-Based Clinical Trials Utilizing *NMR*-Derived Lipoprotein Quantification

Study	CHD Status	CHD Endpoint	*NMR* Associations*
Framingham Offspring Study *2004 AHA*	Primary Prevention	Incident MI, CVA, Claudication or Angina	▲ Total LDL Particles ▲ Small LDL Particles
Women's Health Study *Circ 2002; 106:1930-1937*	Primary Prevention	Incident MI, CHD death, CVA	▲ Total LDL Particles ▲ Small LDL Particles
Cardiovascular Health Study *ATVB 2002; 22:1175-1180*	Primary Prevention	Incident MI or Angina	▲ Total LDL Particles ▲ Small LDL Particles
Healthy Women Study *AJC 2002;90(suppl): 71I-77I*	Primary Prevention	EBCT Coronary Calcium Score	▲ Total LDL Particles ▲ Small LDL Particles ▲ Large VLDL Particles
PLAC-I *AJC 2002;90:89-94*	Secondary Prevention	Angiographic MLD	▲ Total LDL Particles ▲ Small LDL Particles ▼ Large HDL Particles
VA-HDL Intervention Trial *2002 AHA*	Secondary Prevention	Non-Fatal MI or CHD Death	▲ Total LDL Particles ▲ Small LDL Particles ▼ Total HDL Particles

*Significant and independent after multivariate modeling

Image 21: Prospective Outcome-Based Trials Utilizing NMR-Derived Lipoprotein Quantification

The main reason that advanced lipid testing is so currently underutilized is the fact that doctors are human—like everybody else. Some of us are concerned with 'doing the right thing' while others of us are focused on 'doing the easy thing.' Some of us look for reasons and ways to do the right thing while others of us look for excuses why not to do it. Some of us are shepherds while others of us are sheep.

© 1999 Randy Glasbergen.   www.glasbergen.com

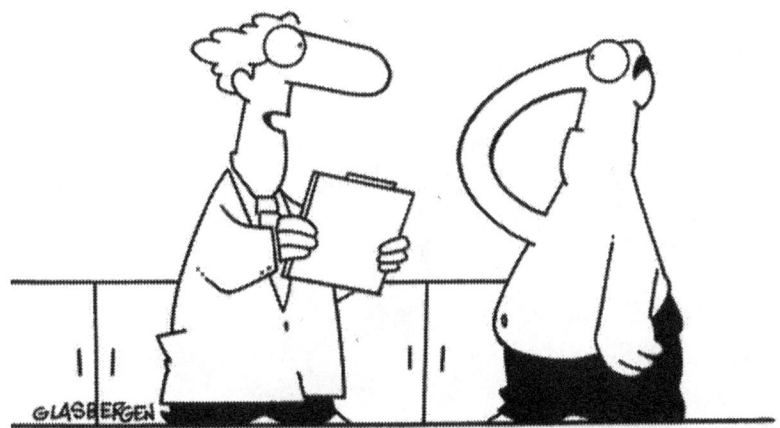

"It's an experimental procedure. Every time you blow your nose, you'll clear out your arteries!"

If you care about your future CV health, you must find a physician who is a passionate shepherd and not one who is a lazy sheep. Please find one who is an early adopter of the truth because there are just way too many late adopters out there. It is crucial to have lipoprotein disorders appropriately diagnosed. If the diagnosis is suspect, the therapy (whether nutritional alone or combined with pharmaceuticals) will <u>NEVER</u> truly be appropriate and/or optimal. In fact, in order for you to utilize the dietary/lifestyle recommendations in this book in the most optimal way possible, it would be very wise to have advanced lipid testing performed to determine whether or not you have increased amounts of large and/or small LDL particles.

If, for whatever reason, you have no access to advanced lipid testing, you could guess the likelihood of large versus small LDL particles based upon your HDL-C and TG levels (see Image 22 below). In the 'average' person, when HDL-C levels are < 60 mg/dL and/or when TG are > 100 mg/dL, the presence of small LDL particles is likely (when HDL-C < 40 mg/dL and/or TG > 150 mg/dL, the predominance of small LDL particles is likely). On the contrary, when HDL-C levels are ≥ 60 mg/dL <u>AND</u> when TG levels are ≤ 100 mg/dL in the 'average' person, the absence of small LDL particles with predominance of large LDL particles is likely. The problem is, no one is an average person—we are all individuals.

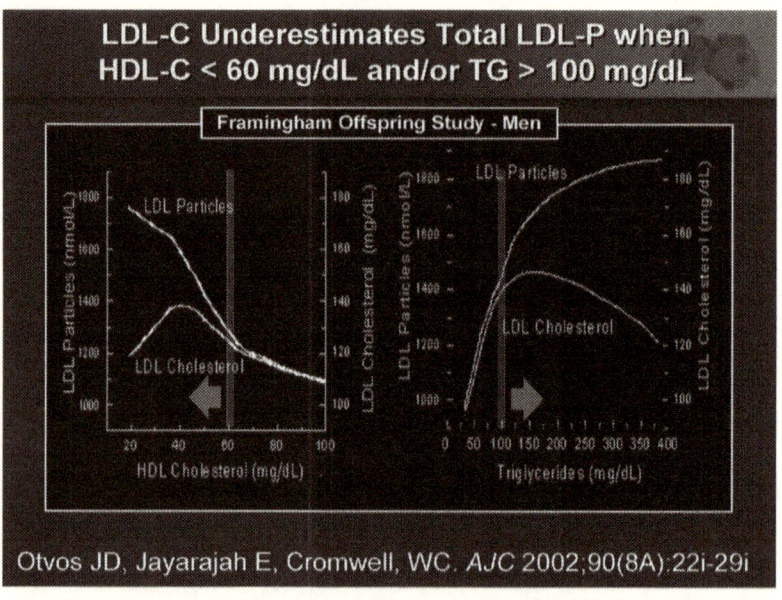

Image 22: LDL-C Underestimates Total LDL-P when
HDL-C < 60 mg/dL and/or TG > 100 mg/dL

I have seen many individual patients with HDL-C levels in the 30s who <u>DID NOT</u> have small LDL particles whereas I have also seen many other individuals with HDL-C levels in the 70s who did not have large LDL particles. The functionality of TG in terms of driving the formation of small, CE-depleted LDL particles and/or HDL-C in terms of maintaining large, CE-enriched LDL particles can not be determined by lipid values. The other problem with guessing based upon HDL-C and TG levels is, even if you're right about the presence or absence of large versus small

LDL particles, you won't know how many of them actually exist (one way you could access this type of information is with another blood test called ApoB that is included in the Berkeley HeartLab panel). And you must have this specific kind of information in order to make (from the physician's perspective) or follow (from the patient's perspective) any specific lifestyle and/or pharmacologic recommendations. So there's really no way around it—you need the kind of detailed lipoprotein information that is <u>ONLY</u> provided by advanced lipid testing.

Medicare (nationally), Medicaid (in certain states) and many private medical insurers now cover advanced lipid testing. Several private insurers still refuse to do so, obviously as a method to enhance their 'bottom line' but at the expense of their enrollees' health. On the next page is a copy of the form letter I use at my own medical practice to convince such uninformed, unwise and basically unethical medical insurers to cover advanced lipid testing (NMR used as an example).

<u>Sample Patient Case #1</u>

Paul is a 35 year-old overweight Caucasian man without significant personal medical history but with a father who had a fatal heart attack at 38 years of age and an older brother who had coronary artery bypass surgery at 40 years of age. His waist circumference is 42 inches. His blood pressure is in the mid 130s over mid 80s. His fasting blood work looks normal except his FBG level is 103 mg/dL, his HDL-C level is 38 mg/dL and his TG level is 163 mg/dL (his calculated LDL-C is 110 mg/dL). Paul's physician informs him he has 'pre-diabetes' and recommends NMR testing. Such testing shows his total LDL-P to be 2047 nmol/L (very high risk) and his small LDL-P to be 1871 (high risk). Paul begins the HAPI Heart Diet with the intent of lowering his total and small LDL particle levels.

Heart Attack Prevention Institute

Michael P. Varveris, MD—Medical Director
280 N. Tamiami Trail—Naples, FL 34102
(239) 261-3988—FAX (239) 261-1022—www.hapi-naples.com

RE: [PATIENT—DOB]

To whom it may concern,

On [DATE], I ordered NMR LipoProfile blood testing on [PATIENT] who is a patient of mine. Such testing is only currently available through LipoScience whose facilities are located in Raleigh, NC. I did this because I required information regarding lipoprotein particle number and particle size only available by NMR testing. NMR-derived lipoprotein testing has proven superior to any form of lipid testing (including direct LDL-C, TC:HDL-C, LDL size and ApoB) in terms of predicting CHD risk in multiple clinical studies (Cardiovascular Health Study[1], Women's Health Study[2], VA-HIT[3], PLAC-1[4], Healthy Women Study[5], Framingham Offspring Study[6]). In fact, NMR-derived total LDL-P and small LDL-P are the ONLY lipid-related parameters that consistently remain significant and independent predictors of CHD risk when modified for other associated clinical parameters (family history, smoking, obesity, lipids, CRP, HgbA1C).

It has been understood since 1967 that "...dyslipidemia can [actually] be translated into dyslipoproteinemia...[7]" and that "...the shift of emphasis to lipoproteins [rather than lipids] offers distinct advantages in the recognition and management of such disorders.[8]"

Since 2002 it has been widely recognized by numerous authorities in cardiovascular medicine that: 1) "...it is now clear that the concentrations of LDL particles, small LDL particles, large HDL particles and large VLDL particles are better indicators of cardiovascular risk than are the elements of the traditional lipid profile;[9]" 2) "...before initiating statin therapy, baseline measurements, including lipid and lipoprotein profiles that will be used to follow the drug's efficacy and safety should be documented;[10]" and 3) "an NMR imaging-based method has become the gold standard for the quantitation of LDL particle size and LDL particle number.[11]"

Thus, I firmly believe that NMR LipoProfile blood testing ordered by me on [DATE] was of 'medical necessity' in my care of [PATIENT].

Sincerely,

Michael P. Varveris, MD

1. *ATVB* 2002; 22:1175–1180
2. Blake GJ et al. *Circ* 2002; 106:1930–1937
3. Otvos JD et al. 2002 AHA
4. Kuller L et al. *AJC* 2002;90:89–94
5. *AJC* 2002;90(suppl):71i-77i
6. Otvos JD et al. 2004 AHA
7. Fredrickson et al. *NEJM.* 1967;276:148
8. Fredrickson et al. *NEJM.* 1967;276:148
9. Kraus WE, et al. *NEJM.* 2002;347:1483–92
10. Pasternak et al. *JACC.* 2002;40(3):567–572
11. Rader DJ. <u>Textbook of Cardiovascular Medicine 2nd ed</u>. 2002. p. 66

Chapter Two

Introduction to the 'HAPI Heart Diet'

Copyright 2005 by Randy Glasbergen.
www.glasbergen.com

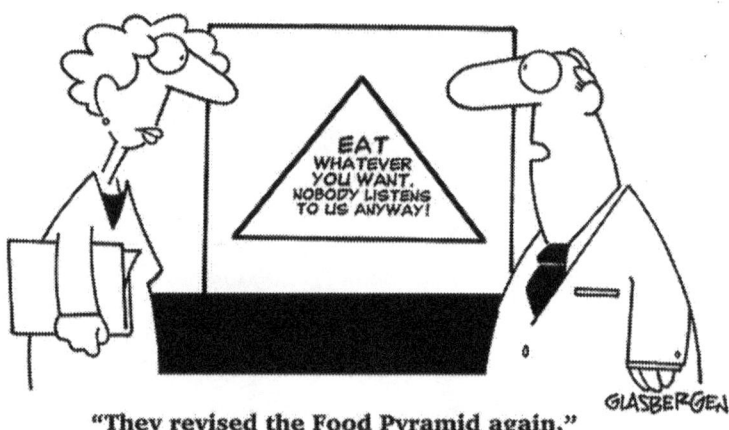

"They revised the Food Pyramid again."

The five main principles of the HAPI Heart Diet are: 1) eat less; 2) eat smarter; 3) exercise more; 4) exercise smarter; and 5) have the right attitude.

In the HAPI Heart Diet, total daily caloric intake must be appropriate to the individual's height and physical activity level. These calories should be consumed in four to six main meals each day, with the largest meals during mid-day. 40–60% of daily calories should come from fat; 20–40%

from carbohydrate; and 20–30% from protein. Less than 1% of daily calories should come from trans fatty acids; less than 10% from omega-6 polyunsaturated fatty acids; and less than 7% from saturated fatty acids.

On the contrary, 20–40% of daily calories should come from omega-9 monounsaturated fatty acids and <u>AT LEAST</u> 1000 mg of marine-derived omega-3 polyunsaturated fatty acids should be consumed every day. Carbohydrates with a relatively low glycemic index (GI) should be eaten throughout the day, except right after exercise, when carbohydrates with a high GI may be eaten. Exercise must be performed each day for at least 60 minutes (preferably in the morning and/or evening) with 60% being aerobic, 20–30% strengthening and 10–20% stretching. Drinking at least six to eight glasses of water (preferably right before as well as in between meals) and adding 25 to 35 grams of supplemental fiber (preferably with meals) is also required. Green/red/white tea should be taken with meals with one to two glasses of red wine (or the equivalent) as an alternative with dinner.

Leafy green vegetables (especially broccoli), cauliflower, peppers, beans, onions, garlic, mushrooms, sweet potatoes, tomatoes, berries, apples, pears, carrots and avocadoes (basically the entire fresh produce section of your local supermarket) should constitute the bulk of the HAPI Heart Diet.

Tree nuts (especially hazelnuts and macadamia nuts) and olive oil should be the main sources of fat (rather than animal fat or other vegetable oils).

Protein should come from legumes and non-fat dairy products such as cottage cheese, yogurt and skim milk. Meat should be eaten only sparingly (four oz serving size—about the size of the four main fingers held together) and should come mainly from fish and shellfish.

Sugars and starches should be eaten but in their natural state (fresh fruits, vegetables and low-fat dairy products) rather than in the form of processed, 'refined' foodstuffs on the HAPI Heart Diet. Whole grain breads, cereals and pastas as well as brown/wild rice can be used, but not excessively. These otherwise healthy carbohydrates should either be taken with your main meals (that also contain protein and fat) along with a fiber supplement or within 30 minutes following exercise.

White bread, white potatoes, white pastas, white rice and white noodles should be avoided. Cookies, cakes, pies, sweets and candies should also be avoided ('just a spoon' after a fine meal on special occasions is OK but please stop at that point). Salt should be avoided while peppers, herbs and spices should be liberally used.

As you can see, the foundation of the HAPI Heart Diet is pursuing a natural lifestyle: being physically active each day and consuming foods at every meal that our bodies were actually designed to consume.

The HAPI Heart Diet is loosely based upon 'The Mediterranean Diet' studied in the Lyon Heart Study. This study involved patients with known coronary heart disease (CHD): a) eating more fresh fruits and vegetables; b) eating more bread and less other starch; c) drinking a modest amount of alcohol; d) eating more fish and less other meat; e) using only olive and canola oil; and f) using no margarine or butter (de Longeril M et al. *Circulation*. 2001:103; 1823–1825). These dietary changes lead to a striking 27% absolute risk reduction (way, way, WAY better than any drug EVER studied for such purposes) in recurrent CV events.

♟

What Foods Should I Consume?

1. Have fresh blueberries and/or blackberries at least once a day. Blueberries and blackberries contain 20 to 50 times more natural antioxidants than other fruits.

2. Have at least two brightly colored fruits or vegetables with each meal. Color indicates the presence of antioxidants and other important phytochemicals: red (cherries, bell peppers, radishes, raspberries, tomatoes); yellow (squash, bell peppers); orange (oranges, carrots, bell peppers); purple (egg plant, red cabbage); and green (spinach, string beans, peas, bell peppers). Although not colored, garlic, onion, shallot and leek should also be used liberally.

3. If eating meat, make fish and/or shellfish your top choice—wild Coho salmon, sea bass, swordfish and bluefin tuna seem most beneficial. Eat on a bed of green lettuce and/or spinach along with fresh tomatoes, carrots and/or red bell peppers.

4. Load your diet with monounsaturated fat by snacking on small handfuls of raw, unsalted tree nuts (almonds, cashews, hazelnuts, macadamia nuts and pecans), using olive oil liberally and avoiding all other cooking oils except macadamia nut and perhaps canola (can take cod liver, herring, salmon and/or sardine oils by the spoonful and use almond, avocado and/or hazelnut oils in vinaigrettes).

♟

What Foods Should I Avoid?

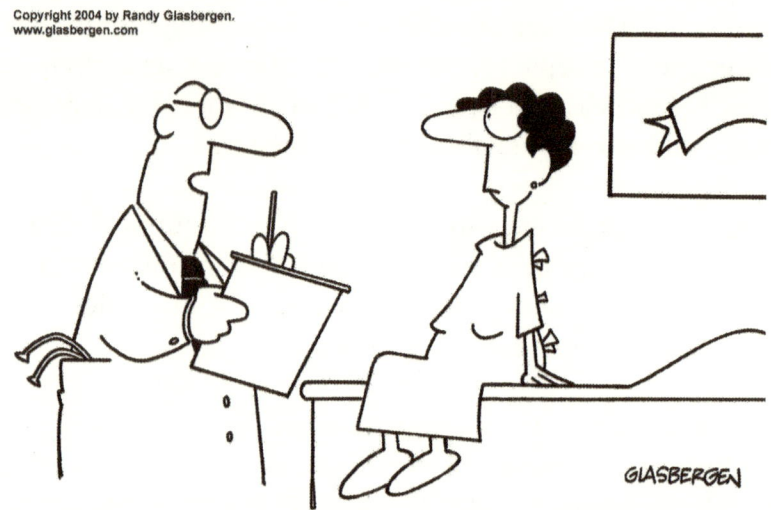

Copyright 2004 by Randy Glasbergen.
www.glasbergen.com

"The 4 Basic Food Groups are: 'don't eat this', 'don't eat that', 'don't eat those' and 'don't eat that other stuff'."

1. Avoid processed, refined high-carbohydrate foods such as white flour, white rice, white potatoes, corn, white pasta, white noodles, white bread, cake, rolls, cookies, crackers, corn chips, potato chips, dough-nuts, cereals, grits, oatmeal, sugar, honey, hard candy, fruit juices and all soft drinks. Also avoid artificial sweeteners. A small amount of dark chocolate (½ oz) each day is probably OK.

2. Avoid legged-animal (non fish) meats (especially poultry and lamb [the latter recommendation causing my soul much pain since I am of Greek descent]). Very infrequently (once or twice per week) may consume small portions of lean non-fish meat (preferably beef or pork tenderloin) for dinner or 99% fat-free turkey breast for sand-wiches (remember to include green lettuce and/or spinach as well as fresh tomato, carrot and/or red bell pepper).

3. Avoid margarines containing trans-or hydrogenated fatty acids.

4. Avoid high-fat milk products especially high-fat, high-salt cheeses and instead consume low-fat/non-fat yogurt, low-fat/non-fat cottage cheese and low-fat/skim milk.

5. Avoid canned foods which are rich in sugar and/or salt (save them for natural disasters—note that frozen foods probably aren't that bad).

6. Eat no more than one whole egg per day—otherwise use Egg Beaters.

Ways to Eat More Vegetables

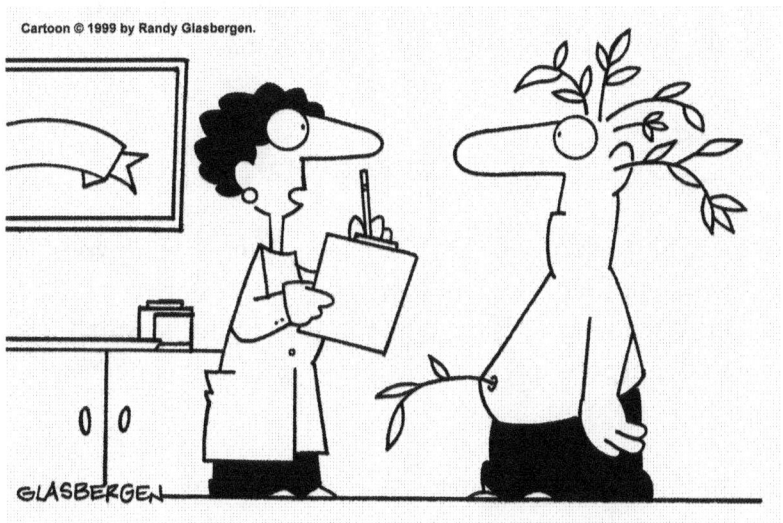

Cartoon © 1999 by Randy Glasbergen.

GLASBERGEN

"It's good that you're eating more fresh fruit and vegetables, but be careful to chew more thoroughly."

1. Rediscover the sweet potato—perhaps the most nutrient-rich fruit or vegetable.

2. Mix three different cans of beans (after rinsing multiple times to remove the salt) with some extra-virgin olive oil, vinegar or fresh lemon juice and spices. Eat this three-bean salad throughout the week.

3. Keep seven bags of your favorite frozen vegetables on hand at all times. Mix any combination, microwave and top with your favorite homemade sauce or salsa. Enjoy 3 to 4 cups a day. Makes a nutritious and quick dinner.

4. Use pre-bagged baby spinach everywhere: as 'lettuce' in sandwiches, heated in soups, wilted in hot whole grain pasta, place under your fish as a 'bed' and added to your salads.

5. Jazz up your vegetables to make them yummy: dribble some molasses or honey over carrots and sprinkle some chopped raw almonds, hazelnuts or macadamia nuts on green beans.

Δ

Great Places to Start

1. Make eating purposeful, not mindless. After plating your food, sit down, cut the food into bite-sized portions (staring at the food as you cut it) and bring it to your mouth (trying to smell it), slowly chew and purposefully swallow. Engage all of your senses in the nourishment of your body.

2. Start the day with a good breakfast. It will help you to eat fewer total calories later in the day.

3. Drink at least six to eight 8-oz glasses of water per day—one to two in the AM right after awakening, one right before each meal and one in the PM before going to sleep.

4. Drink one cup of green, red or white tea with each main meal—can instead consume one to two alcoholic drinks (5 oz glass of wine, 3 oz glass of fortified wine [such as Madeira, Port and/or Sherry], 12 oz bottle of beer or an ounce of 80-proof distilled liquor) with main evening meal.

5. Take one to two Fiber Choice sugar-free wafers at the beginning of each main meal. Remember to add fiber to your diet gradually to prevent bloating, gas, diarrhea and abdominal discomfort.

Dr. V's Pyramid to a HAPI Heart

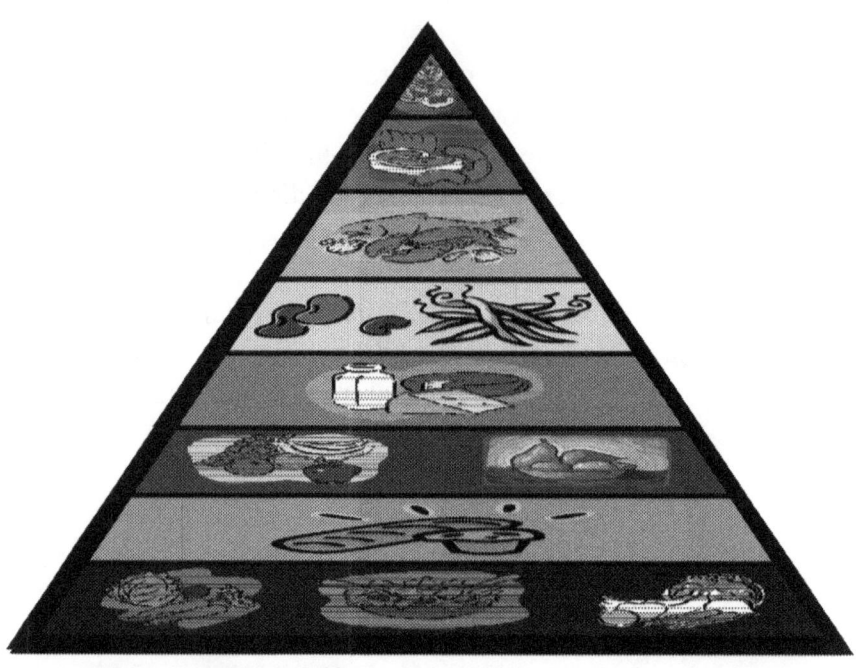

LEGGED-ANIMAL MEATS – Eat ≤ 1 egg per day and ≤ two 4-6 oz servings of lean beef, lamb, pork, poultry, veal and/or venison per week	**REFINED CARBOHYDRATES** – Avoid processed sugars/starches (sweets, 'junk' snackfoods, white flour, white bread, white rice, white pasta, etc…)
BEANS/LEGUMES – Eat 2-3 cups of dried beans, peas and/or lentils every day	**FISH/SHELLFISH** – Eat 4-6 oz of fresh/frozen fish and/or shellfish every day – use olive/canola oils only
FRUITS/NUTS – Eat 2-3 cups of fresh fruit (especially berries) and 1-2 oz of raw tree nuts every day	**DAIRY** – Get 2-3 cups of low-fat milk, yogurt or cottage cheese every day – avoid cream/butter/margarine
VEGETABLES – Eat 3-4 cups of fresh/frozen vegetables (especially dark green and orange) every day	**WHOLE GRAINS** – Eat 3-4 cups of whole grains (bread, cereal, pasta) or brown/wild rice every day

♖

Chapter Three
HAPI Diet Principle #1: 'Eat Less'

Copyright 2003 by Randy Glasbergen.
www.glasbergen.com

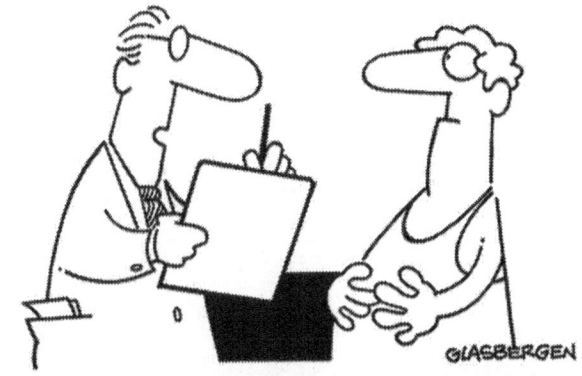

"I understand how difficult it is to lose weight, so
we're going to staple your stomach. Then we're
going to duct tape it, glue it, paperclip it, tie it
up with rope, surround it with barbed wire...."

♙

Consume Fewer Calories Each & Every Day

The whole trick to losing weight is to have a negative caloric balance
on a day by day basis (i.e. less calories coming into the body from foodstuffs than are being burned off by exercise and the basal metabolic rate

[BMR] of the body). This obviously begins by consuming fewer calories. You <u>MUST</u> count your calories—at least for the first few weeks or so.

Counting calories will serve two main purposes: 1) you will learn what particular foods contain what number of calories so you can realize which caloric-rich foods to avoid; and 2) you will get an idea of what your average daily caloric intake really is in order to make the appropriate lifestyle changes with at least some semblance of objectivity. You should decrease your caloric intake by at least 500 calories per day.

Food	Serving Size	Calories	Protein (g)	Fat (g)	Carb (g)	Fiber (g)
Almonds	1 oz	164	6	14	6	3
Apple	1 item	81	0	1	21	4
Apple butter	1 T.	37	0	0	9	0
Apple juice	1 cup	117	0	0	29	0
Applesauce	½ cup	53	0	0	14	1
Apricot	3 items	51	1	0	12	3
Apricot nectar	½ cup	71	0	0	18	1
Artichoke, globe	½ cup	51	4	1	10	5
Artichoke, Jerusalem	1 cup	114	3	0	26	2
Asparagus	1 cup	31	3	0	6	3
Avocado	½ cup	185	2	18	9	6
Bacon	1 slice	44	3	3	0	0
Banana	1 item	105	1	1	27	3
Barley	1 cup	651	23	4	135	32
Bass, striped	4 oz	140	26	3	0	0
Bass, fresh-water	4 oz	165	27	5	0	0
Baked beans	1 cup	236	12	1	52	13
Beans, green	1 cup	44	2	0	10	4
Beans, kidney	1 cup	225	15	1	40	13
Beans, lima	1 cup	229	15	1	42	14

Food	Serving Size	Calories	Protein (g)	Fat (g)	Carb (g)	Fiber (g)
Beans, navy	1 cup	109	7	0	19	5
Bean sprouts	1 cup	31	3	0	6	2
Beef, lean, ground	3 oz	224	15	18	0	0
Beef, rib roast	3 oz	291	19	23	0	0
Beef, round roast	3 oz	161	25	6	0	0
Beef, tenderloin	4 oz	218	32	9	0	0
Beer	12 oz	146	1	0	13	1
Beets	1 cup	54	2	0	12	4
Benecol, Light	1 T.	50	0	5	0	0
Blackberries	1 cup	75	1	1	18	8
Blueberries	1 cup	81	1	1	21	4
Bison (sirloin)	4 oz	193	32	6	0	0
Bran, oat	1 cup	276	15	5	4	13
Bratwurst	1 item	286	12	27	0	0
Brazil nuts	1 oz	186	4	19	3	2
Bread, rye	1 slice	83	3	1	16	2
Bread, white	1 slice	67	2	1	12	1
Bread, wheat	1 slice	62	2	1	12	2
Broccoli	1 cup	25	3	0	5	3
Brussels sprouts	1 cup	87	7	1	18	8
Butter, unsalted	1 T.	102	0	11	0	0
Cabbage	1 cup	18	1	0	4	2
Cake, angel	2 oz slice	146	3	0	33	1
Cake, pound	2 oz slice	219	3	11	28	0
Calamari	3 oz	78	13	1	0	0
Canola oil	1 T.	124	0	14	0	0
Cantaloupe	1 item	392	11	1	98	14
Caramels	2 items	43	0	0	10	0
Carrots, cooked	1 cup	70	2	0	16	5
Carrots, raw	1 cup	31	1	0	7	2

Food	Serving Size	Calories	Protein (g)	Fat (g)	Carb (g)	Fiber (g)
Cashew nuts	1 oz	157	5	12	9	1
Catfish	4 oz	119	21	3	0	0
Cauliflower	1 cup	29	2	1	5	3
Caviar	1 T.	40	4	3	1	0
Celery	2 stalks	13	1	0	3	1
Cereal, raisin bran	1 cup	170	5	1	43	7
Cheese, American	1 oz	105	6	9	0	0
Cheese, Camembert	1 oz	85	6	7	0	0
Cheese, Cheddar	1 oz	113	7	9	0	0
Cheese, cottage	1 cup	123	25	1	3	0
Cheese, cream, regular	1 T.	51	1	5	0	0
Cheese, cream, low fat	1 T.	35	2	3	1	0
Cheese, Parmesan	1 T.	23	2	2	0	0
Cheese, ricotta	1 cup	360	28	24	12	0
Cheese, Roquefort	1 oz	103	6	9	1	0
Cheese, Swiss	1 oz	105	8	8	1	0
Cherries	15 items	74	1	1	17	2
Chicken, dark meat, roasted	3.5 oz	203	27	10	0	0
Chicken breast, skin-less, roasted	4 oz	186	35	4	0	0
Chickpeas	1 cup	509	21	21	62	16
Chocolate, bittersweet	1 oz	138	2	10	16	2
Chocolate, milk	1 oz	153	2	9	16	1
Chocolate fudge	1 piece	65	0	1	14	0
Chocolate syrup	1 T.	51	0	0	12	1

Food	Serving Size	Calories	Protein (g)	Fat (g)	Carb (g)	Fiber (g)
Clams, raw	3 oz	63	11	1	2	0
Cocoa mix, powdered	2 oz	206	6	2	45	1
Coconut	1 cup	283	3	27	12	7
Cod, Atlantic	4 oz	119	26	1	0	0
Coffee	1 cup	5	0	0	1	0
Collard greens	1 cup	61	5	1	12	5
Corn ear, cooked	1 item	83	3	1	19	2
Corn oil	1 T.	120	0	14	0	0
Corn flakes	1 cup	110	2	0	26	1
Cornmeal	1 cup	212	3	1	26	2
Cornstarch	1 cup	488	0	0	117	1
Crab meat	4 oz	95	21	1	0	0
Crab, king	1 leg	130	26	2	0	0
Cracker, Graham	1 item	30	0	1	5	0
Cracker, saltine	1 item	13	0	0	2	0
Cranberries	1 cup	54	0	0	14	5
Cream, half-and-half	1 T.	20	0	2	1	0
Cream, sour, regular	1 T.	26	0	3	1	0
Cream, sour, low fat	1 T.	20	0	2	1	0
Cream, whipping, heavy	1 T.	52	1	6	1	0
Cream, whipping, light	1 T.	44	1	5	1	0
Cucumber	1 cup	14	1	0	3	1
Dates	3 items	72	1	0	19	2
Doughnut, glazed	1 item	192	2	10	23	1
Dressing, Thousand Island	1 T.	59	0	6	2	0

Food	Serving Size	Calories	Protein (g)	Fat (g)	Carb (g)	Fiber (g)
Dressing, French	1 T.	67	0	6	3	0
Duck breast, roasted skinless	4 oz	158	31	3	0	0
Egg, whole, poached	1 item	78	6	5	1	0
Egg yolk	1 item	59	3	5	0	0
Egg white	1 item	17	4	0	0	0
Eggplant	1 cup	21	1	0	5	2
Endive	1 cup	9	1	0	2	2
English muffin	1 item	134	4	1	26	2
Fig	1 item	37	0	0	10	2
Flaxseed, ground	1 T.	37	1	3	2	2
Flounder	4 oz	132	27	2	0	0
Flour, cake	1 cup	395	9	1	85	2
Flour, rye	1 cup	231	29	12	0	0
Flour, whole wheat	1 cup	407	16	2	87	15
Flour, white	1 cup	420	12	1	88	3
Flounder	3.4 oz	133	21	5	0	0
Frankfurter	1 item	88	6	6	1	0
Frog legs	1 cup	165	37	1	0	0
Gelatin, plain	1 cup	142	4	0	34	0
Gin	4 oz	257	0	0	0	0
Ginger, raw	1 cup	66	2	1	15	2
Ginger ale	12 oz	125	0	0	32	0
Grape juice	1 cup	154	1	0	38	0
Grapefruit	1 item	118	3	1	29	18
Grapefruit juice	1 cup	94	1	0	22	0
Grapes, seedless	1 cup	58	1	0	16	1
Grits	1 cup	145	3	0	32	0
Grouper	4 oz	133	28	2	0	0

Food	Serving Size	Calories	Protein (g)	Fat (g)	Carb (g)	Fiber (g)
Guava	1 item	46	1	1	11	5
Haddock	4 oz	127	27	1	0	0
Halibut	4 oz	158	30	3	0	0
Hamburger	1 item	140	22	5	0	0
Ham, lean	3 oz	134	21	5	0	0
Hazelnuts	1 oz	178	4	17	5	3
Herring, Atlantic	4 oz	229	26	13	0	0
Hollandaise sauce	1 T.	80	1	7	3	0
Honey	1 T.	74	0	0	17	0
Honeydew	1 cup	60	1	0	16	1
Horseradish	1 T.	13	0	0	3	0
Ice cream, chocolate, regular	½ cup	143	3	7	19	0
Ice cream, chocolate, rich	½ cup	189	4	13	15	0
Ice cream, chocolate, low fat	½ cup	135	3	5	20	0
Ice cream, vanilla, regular	½ cup	145	3	8	17	0
Ice cream, vanilla, rich	½ cup	266	4	17	24	0
Ice cream, vanilla, light	½ cup	125	4	4	20	0
Jam	1 T.	48	0	0	13	0
Kale	1 cup	42	2	1	7	3
Ketchup	1 T.	16	0	0	4	0
Kiwi	1 item	46	1	0	11	3
Kumquat	1 item	12	0	0	3	1
Lamb loin chop	4 oz	228	30	12	0	0
Lamb shank	3 oz	191	22	11	0	0
Lard	1 T.	115	0	13	0	0

Food	Serving Size	Calories	Protein (g)	Fat (g)	Carb (g)	Fiber (g)
Leek	1 item	76	2	0	18	2
Lemon	1 item	22	1	0	12	5
Lentils	1 oz	90	5	0	17	2
Lettuce, iceberg	1 head	120	6	1	21	9
Lime	1 item	20	0	0	7	2
Liverwurst	1 slice	59	3	5	0	0
Lobster	1 cup	204	43	2	1	0
Lobster, northern	4 oz	108	23	1	1	0
Macadamia nuts	1 oz	204	2	21	4	2
Macaroni	1 cup	155	5	1	32	2
Mackerel, Atlantic	4 oz	296	27	20	0	0
Mango	1 item	135	1	1	35	4
Maple syrup	1 T.	48	0	0	12	0
Margarine	1 T.	101	0	11	0	0
Marmalade	1 oz	67	0	0	17	0
Marshmallows	5 items	115	1	0	29	0
Mayonnaise	1 T.	100	0	11	0	0
Melba toast	1 slice	16	1	0	3	0
Buttermilk	1 cup	59	4	0	13	7
Milk, 1%	1 cup	102	8	3	12	0
Milk, 2%	1 cup	121	8	5	12	0
Milk, chocolate	1 cup	193	7	7	26	1
Milk, skim	1 cup	86	8	0	12	0
Milk, whole	1 cup	150	8	8	11	0
Molasses	1 cup	44	0	0	11	0
Muffin, corn	1 item	174	3	5	29	2
Mushrooms	1 cup	18	1	0	3	1
Mustard greens	1 cup	21	3	0	3	3
Nectarine	1 item	67	1	1	16	2
Noodles, egg	1 cup	213	8	2	40	2

Food	Serving Size	Calories	Protein (g)	Fat (g)	Carb (g)	Fiber (g)
Oatmeal, instant	1 cup	145	6	2	25	4
Okra	1 cup	32	2	0	7	3
Oil, almond	1 T.	124	0	14	0	0
Oil, avocado	1 T.	124	0	14	0	0
Oil, coconut	1 T.	117	0	14	0	0
Oil, cod liver	1 T.	123	0	14	0	0
Oil, corn	1 T.	120	0	14	0	0
Oil, flaxseed	1 T.	120	0	14	0	0
Oil, grapeseed	1 T.	120	0	14	0	0
Oil, hazelnut	1 T.	120	0	14	0	0
Oil, herring	1 T.	123	0	14	0	0
Oil, macadamia nut	1 T.	123	0	14	0	0
Oil, olive	1 T.	119	0	14	0	0
Oil, palm	1 T.	120	0	14	0	0
Oil, palm kernel	1 T.	117	0	14	0	0
Oil, peanut	1 T.	120	0	14	0	0
Oil, primrose	1 T.	120	0	14	0	0
Oil, safflower	1 T.	120	0	14	0	0
Oil, salmon	1 T.	123	0	14	0	0
Oil, sardine	1 T.	123	0	14	0	0
Oil, sesame	1 T.	120	0	14	0	0
Oil, soybean	1 T.	104	0	14	0	0
Oil, sunflower	1 T.	120	0	14	0	0
Oil, walnut	1 T.	120	0	14	0	0
Olives	1 large	10	0	1	1	0
Onion	1 cup	61	2	0	14	3
Orange	1 item	62	1	0	15	3
Orange juice	1 cup	112	2	1	26	1
Oysters	1 cup	134	12	4	13	0
Papaya	1 cup	55	1	0	14	3

Food	Serving Size	Calories	Protein (g)	Fat (g)	Carb (g)	Fiber (g)
Parsley	1 T.	1	0	0	0	0
Parsnips	1 cup	113	2	0	27	6
Peach	1 item	37	1	0	10	2
Peanut butter	1 T.	95	4	8	3	1
Peanuts	1 oz	168	5	15	7	3
Pear	1 item	98	1	1	25	4
Peas, black-eyed	1 cup	561	39	2	100	18
Peas, green	1 cup	134	9	0	25	9
Peas, split	1 cup	231	16	1	41	16
Pecans	1 oz	196	3	20	4	3
Pepper, chili	1 item	10	0	0	2	1
Pepper, green	1 item	25	2	0	5	3
Pepperoni	1 slice	27	1	2	0	0
Pickle, dill	1 item	12	0	0	3	0
Pineapple	1 cup	76	1	1	19	2
Pine nuts	1 oz	191	4	19	4	1
Pistachios	1 oz	162	6	13	8	3
Plum	1 item	105	2	2	38	4
Pomegranate	1 item	105	1	0	26	1
Popcorn	1 cup	40	1	1	8	1
Pork chop	3 oz	197	24	11	0	0
Pork tenderloin	4 oz	211	34	7	0	0
Potato, baked	1 item	220	5	0	51	5
Potato, boiled	1 cup	212	5	0	49	4
Pretzels, thin	5 items	5	0	0	1	0
Prunes	1 cup	339	4	1	88	10
Pumpkin	1 cup	30	1	0	8	1
Rabbit, roasted	4 oz	171	25	7	0	0
Radishes	3 items	2	0	0	0	0
Raisins	1 cup	435	5	1	115	6
Raspberries	1 cup	60	1	1	14	8

Food	Serving Size	Calories	Protein (g)	Fat (g)	Carb (g)	Fiber (g)
Red snapper	3 oz	109	22	1	0	0
Rhubarb	1 cup	513	3	16	96	4
Rice, brown, cooked	1 cup	218	5	2	46	4
Rice, white, cooked	1 cup	242	4	0	53	1
Rice, wild, cooked	1 cup	166	7	1	35	3
Roll, white	2 oz	167	6	2	30	1
Root beer	12 oz	151	0	0	39	0
Rum	4 oz	257	0	0	0	0
Salami	1 oz	115	6	10	0	0
Salmon, Atlantic, wild	4 oz	262	29	9	0	0
Sardines, canned in oil	3 oz	206	29	10	0	0
Sauerkraut	1 cup	20	0	0	4	4
Sausage, link	1 item	80	9	7	0	0
Scallop, large	1 item	26	5	0	1	0
Sea Bass	4 oz	140	27	3	0	0
Seeds, pumpkin	1 oz	148	9	12	4	1
Seeds, sunflower	1 oz	165	5	14	7	3
Shark	4 oz	147	24	5	0	0
Sherbet	1 cup	270	2	4	59	0
Sherry, dry	4 oz	159	0	0	9	0
Shrimp, boiled	3 oz	84	18	1	0	0
Smart Balance, Light	1 T.	47	0	9	0	0
Smart Balance, Omega Plus	1 T.	85	0	5	0	0
Snapper	4 oz	145	30	2	0	0
Sole	1 piece	149	31	2	0	0

Food	Serving Size	Calories	Protein (g)	Fat (g)	Carb (g)	Fiber (g)
Soybeans	1 cup	197	7	1	40	2
Spaghetti, cooked	1 cup	197	7	1	40	2
Spareribs, roasted	3 oz	208	24	12	0	0
Spinach	1 cup	12	2	0	2	2
Squash, boiled	1 cup	29	1	0	8	3
Squash, butternut, baked	1 cup	82	2	0	22	7
Strawberries	1 cup	45	1	0	11	3
Sugar, brown	1 cup	827	0	0	214	0
Sugar, white	1 cup	774	0	0	200	0
Swordfish	4 oz	175	29	6	0	0
Taco shell	1 item	61	1	3	8	1
Tangerine	1 item	37	1	0	9	2
Tartar sauce	1 T.	76	0	8	1	0
Tea	1 cup	2	0	0	0	0
Tilapia	4 oz	145	30	3	0	0
Tilefish	4 oz	166	28	5	0	0
Tofu, firm	8 oz	329	36	20	10	5
Tofu, soft	8 oz	122	11	7	5	0
Tomato, raw	1 item	26	1	0	6	1
Tomato juice	1 cup	40	2	0	10	2
Tomatoes, canned	1 cup	46	2	0	11	2
Tortilla	1 item	56	1	1	12	1
Trout, rainbow, wild	3 oz	169	26	7	0	0
Tuna, canned in oil	3 oz	158	22	7	0	0
Tuna, canned in water	3 oz	109	20	1	0	0
Tuna, yellowtail	4 oz	157	34	1	0	0

Food	Serving Size	Calories	Protein (g)	Fat (g)	Carb (g)	Fiber (g)
Turkey breast, skinless, roasted	4 oz	153	34	1	0	0
Turkey, dark meat	1 cup	262	40	10	0	0
Turnips	1 cup	39	2	0	11	4
Vanilla extract	1 T.	44	0	0	4	0
Veal chop	4 oz	198	30	8	0	0
Veal sirloin	3 oz	143	22	5	0	0
Venison tenderloin	4 oz	168	34	3	0	0
Vodka	4 oz	257	0	0	0	0
Walnuts	1 oz	185	4	18	4	2
Watercress	1 cup	4	1	0	0	1
Watermelon	1 cup	51	1	1	12	1
Wheat germ	1 T.	26	2	1	4	1
Whiskey	4 oz	257	0	0	0	0
Whitefish	3 oz	146	21	6	0	0
Wine, dry	5 oz	149	0	0	1	0
Yams	1 cup	158	2	0	38	5
Yeast, brewers	1 T.	25	3	0	3	3
Yeast, compressed	1 oz	24	3	0	3	2
Yogurt, full-fat, plain	1 cup	139	8	7	11	0
Yogurt, nonfat, plain	1 cup	133	13	0	19	0
Zucchini	1 cup	29	1	0	7	3

Table 1: Caloric Composition of Foods

Starvation is obviously quite harmful to the body so don't consume less than 1200 calories per day if you are a woman and don't consume less than 1500 calories per day if you are a man. Other than causing obvious health problems, short-term starvation (relatively speaking) can actually be counter-productive long-term on a weight loss plan. The human body (like all natural entities) follows the principle of balance or 'homeostasis.' When your caloric intake is insufficient to fuel the demands of normal body metabolism, your BMR will slow down as a response in order to return to a state of homeostasis.

Copyright 2001 by Randy Glasbergen. www.glasbergen.com

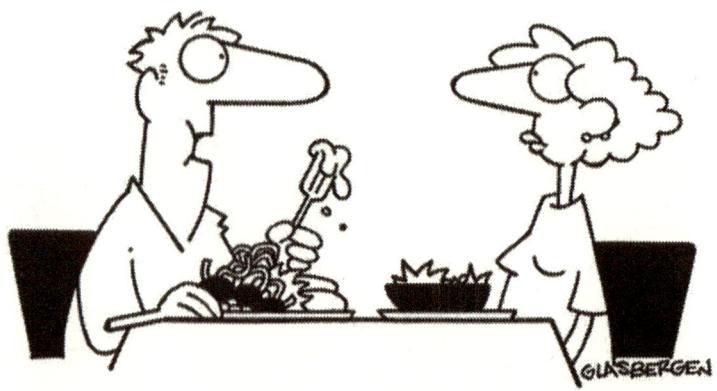

"If God wanted us to count calories, He would have put calculator buttons on our tongues."

A good way to determine the appropriate number of calories for you to consume each day is first to calculate your ideal body weight (IBW— see Tables 2 and 3 below). Obviously this is a very crude way of estimating IBW (due to significant individual variability in bone and muscle mass) but it should suffice. Weight within 10–15% of IBW is considered 'normal.' Weight > 20% but < 30% of IBW is considered 'overweight.' Weight ≥ 30% of IBW is considered 'obese.'

Next, you need to get a sense of your overall daily activity level (not including your daily exercise—see Table 4 below). I would recommend you consider purchasing an electronic pedometer (basic models costing around $10) for this purpose. 10,000 steps per day is basically the equivalent of 60 minutes of 'extra' aerobic exercise as well as being close to five miles. 'Tricks' to increase your daily walking include: 1) parking your car further away from the entrance to the shopping center or your office; 2) using the stairs rather than the elevator; 3) taking frequent rest stops on long car trips in order to walk for 15 minutes or so; 4) taking a walk instead of just killing time waiting for an appointment; and 5) taking your dog on more frequent walks (if you don't have a dog, consider getting one).

As you can see in Table 4, multiplying your IBW by a daily activity modifier (ten to 15) determines the baseline amount of calories you get to consume each day. Again, this is rather simplistic but does make sense and is a good place to start. Distribute these calories over four to six meals each day with the largest meals during mid-day. You can add to this baseline the number of calories expended during your daily exercise—these calories should be consumed within 30 minutes following your exercise at a 'post-workout meal.'

Height	IBW
5'4"	130
5'5"	136
5'6"	142
5'7"	148
5'8"	154
5'9"	160
5'10"	166
5'11"	172
6'0"	178
6'1"	184
6'2"	190

Table 2. IBW for Men

Height	IBW
5'0"	105
5'1"	110
5'2"	115
5'3"	120
5'4"	125
5'5"	130
5'6"	135
5'7"	140
5'8"	145
5'9"	150
5'10"	155

Table 3. IBW for Women

Daily Activity Level	Number of Steps	Total Daily Calories
Very Sedentary	< 1000	IBW times 10
Moderately Sedentary	1000–2999	IBW times 11
Somewhat Active	3000–5000	IBW times 12
Moderately Active	5001–9999	IBW times 13
Very Active	10,000–15,000	IBW times 14
Very, Very Active	> 15,000	IBW times 15

Table 4. Baseline Daily Calorie Calculation

Sample Patient Case #2

Lisa is a 47 year-old overweight Caucasian woman with high blood pressure and mild arthritis in her knees. She is 5'6" tall and weighs 165 pounds. She decides to begin the HAPI Heart Diet. She purchases a pedometer and, after one week of use, determines she walks about 3500–4000 steps per day. She estimates her IBW at 135 (±13–14) pounds and thus decides to cut her daily calories to about 1600–1700. Lisa separates these calories over four to six main meals each day, with the largest meals in the afternoon and early evening.

Tips on Cutting Calories

1. Leave 1/3 of each item on your plate, wait until your cravings have disappeared (usually within 10 minutes—you'll know it's time when you bring each item from the plate to your mouth, the thought of actually putting it into your mouth, chewing and swallowing seems almost revolting) THEN throw the remaining food away in the trash. Since all our mothers taught us not to waste food, this will force us

over time to develop good eating habits (eating smaller meals, eating more slowly and eating more frequently).

2. <u>NEVER</u> have seconds.

3. Follow the Chinese proverb: "Eat until you are eight-tenths full."

4. Use a salad plate instead of a dinner plate.

5. <u>NEVER</u> super-size your food portions—unless you want to super-size your clothes.

6. Eat the low-cal items on your plate first and then graduate. Start with salads, vegetables and broth soups, eating meats and starches last. When you get to them, you'll be full enough to be content with smaller portions of those high-cal, high-fat and/or high-GI items.

7. <u>NEVER</u> eat right before you take a nap or go to sleep.

8. Keep a food journal.

9. Cut out all high-cal, sugar-loaded drinks such as soda, sweet tea, Gatorade, lemonade, etc.

10. Take your own 'bagged' lunch to work.

11. Eat at home rather than going out to eat.

12. When eating out, 'halve it' and bag the rest for tomorrow's lunch or dinner. A typical restaurant entrée will have 1,000 to 2,000 calories.

13. When eating out, never take more than a bite or two of any bread, rolls or chips while you wait for your order to arrive.

14. When eating out, order only one dessert to share.

15. Get calories from foods you chew rather than beverages. Have fresh fruit and vegetables (with their skins—if edible) instead of fruit or vegetable juice.

16. See what you plan to eat. Plate your food instead of eating right from the jar or bag.

17. Sit down when you eat.

18. Eat a small amount of fresh, raw food (celery, carrot, cucumber) right before your meal and another small amount of fresh, raw food (parsley, apple, banana) right after your meal.

19. Mix one tablespoon pure apple cider vinegar in an 8-oz glass of water and drink this right before each main meal.

20. Get enough B vitamins, vitamin C, calcium and potassium in your diet (from natural foods and/or dietary supplements).

21. Use mustard rather than mayo.

22. Eat more homemade soup.

23. Dilute fruit and vegetable juice 50:50 with water.

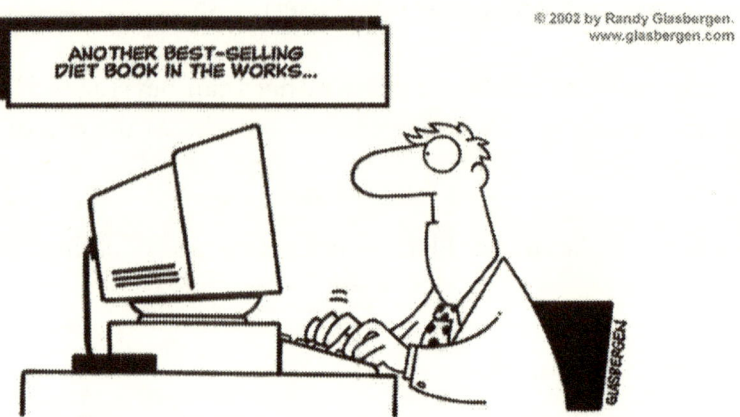

"Diet Tip #97: Eat a pint of ice cream to reduce your craving for sweets. Diet Tip #98: To melt your waistline, eat your pizza very, very hot. Diet Tip #99: Chewing burns more calories than not chewing..."

Pitfalls to Avoid

1. Skipping meals. Many otherwise healthy eaters 'diet' during the day but then 'binge' at night.

2. Don't 'graze' yourself into becoming fat. You can easily pig out on 600 calories of pretzels, chips or cereal without even realizing it.

3. Ignoring 'Serving Size' information on the Nutrition Facts panel. One simple option is to use those natural measuring devices given to you by the Creator (your hands)—your thumb is a good estimate for servings of avocadoes, cheese, olives and nut butters; your four main fingers held together for meat or bread; your palm for cottage cheese and egg; your cupped hand for dry whole grains, nuts and seeds; and your closed fist for fruits, vegetables, potatoes, beans, yogurt and cooked noodles/pasta/rice.

Chapter Four
HAPI Diet Principle #2: 'Eat Smarter'

Copyright 2002 by Randy Glasbergen.
www.glasbergen.com

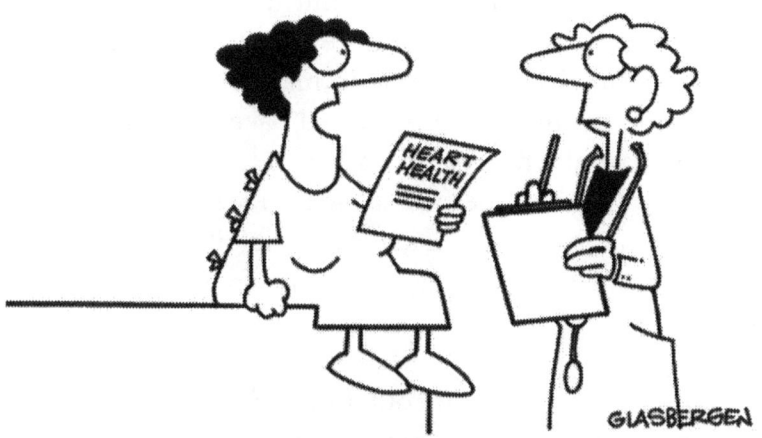

"First you put me on a low-fat diet, then you tell me
to eat more oily fish — MAKE UP YOUR MIND!"

Part I. Fat

Fats should constitute 40–60% of your total daily calories on the HAPI Heart Diet. Fats contain nine calories per gram (compared to protein and carbohydrate which each contain four calories per gram). Energy is stored in the body mostly in the form of fat. Fat is needed in the diet to supply essential fatty acids, substances necessary for proper body functioning but not produced by the body itself. Each of your four to six main meals per day should contain a balanced amount of fat in relationship to protein and carbohydrate. However, your post-workout meal(s) should contain very little, if any, fat.

♟

Trans Fats are VERY Bad

Trans fatty acids (TFAs) can increase the production of both large as well as small LDL particles (increasing LDL-C and decreasing HDL-C). The most common TFA is elaidic acid (the trans isomer of oleic acid, an otherwise beneficial omega-9 monounsaturated fatty acid described below). The structure of elaidic acid is much straighter than oleic acid such that the former can be packed more tightly to assume a solid form at room temperature. TFAs are found in margarines, shortenings, milk, butter, cheese and commercially processed baked goods. Any foodstuff that mentions "partially hydrogenated" (a code phrase for TFA) in the ingredients section should best be avoided. Please note that fast-food restaurants commonly use TFA-rich vegetable oils. You should get less than one percent of your total daily calories from TFAs on the HAPI Heart Diet.

One ounce of corn chips can contain up to 1.5 grams of TFAs; one tablespoon of soft tub margarine up to 2 grams; one tablespoon of vegetable shortening, one average-size Danish pastry, three cups of microwave popcorn or six frozen fish sticks up to 3 grams; one tablespoon of stick margarine up to 3.5 grams; five ounces of frozen fries up to 4 grams; and 1 medium-size frozen pot pie up to 16 grams.

♟

Excess Omega-6 Fats are Bad

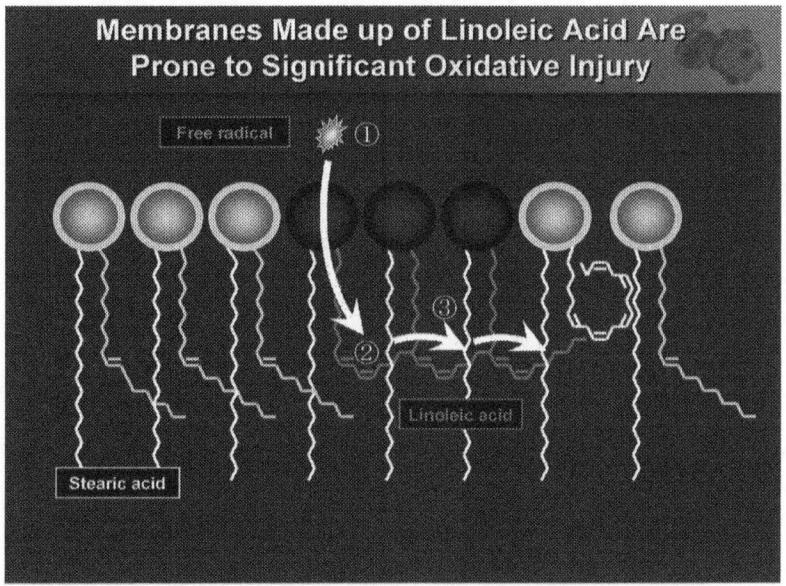

Image 23: Membranes Made up of Linoleic Acid Are
Prone to Significant Oxidative Injury

Omega-6 polyunsaturated fatty acids (ω-6 PUFAs) enhance tissue oxidation (see Image 23 above) as well as inflammation (processes involved with CV disease, type II DM, MS/IR, obesity, arthritis, asthma, allergies, autoimmune disease, cancer and the aging process) and thus increase small LDL particle concentrations (decreasing both LDL-C and HDL-C—see Image 24 below). The most common ω-6 PUFA is linoleic acid. Omega-6 PUFAs are found in high concentrations in seed oils and soft margarines. They are also found in all meat products to a lesser extent (lowest amount in fish and highest amount in poultry). Note that ω-6 PUFAs are essential fatty acids (necessary for various metabolic processes but not produced by the body) and thus a diet entirely devoid of them is unhealthy. You should, however, get less than ten percent of your total daily calories from ω-6 PUFAs.

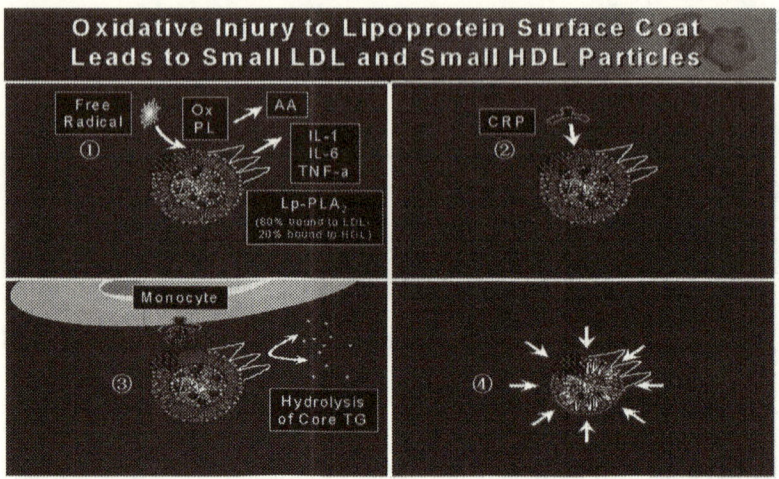

Image 24: Oxidative Injury to Lipoprotein Surface Coat
Leads to Small LDL and Small HDL Particles

♙

Saturated Fats and Dietary Cholesterol are Bad

Saturated fatty acids (SFAs) and dietary cholesterol can increase large LDL particle levels (increasing LDL-C). High concentrations of SFAs are found in fatty non-fish meats, high-fat dairy products and certain vegetable oils such as coconut, palm and palm kernel oil. Dietary cholesterol is found in all animal products including fish and shellfish. Cutting back on SFAs seems more important than cutting back on dietary cholesterol in overweight people as well as in Caucasians while cutting back on dietary cholesterol seems just as important as cutting back on SFAs in slender people and in non-Caucasians. You should get less than seven percent of your total calories from SFAa and no more than 300 mg of dietary cholesterol each day on the HAPI Heart Diet.

♟

Marine-Derived Omega-3 Fats are Good

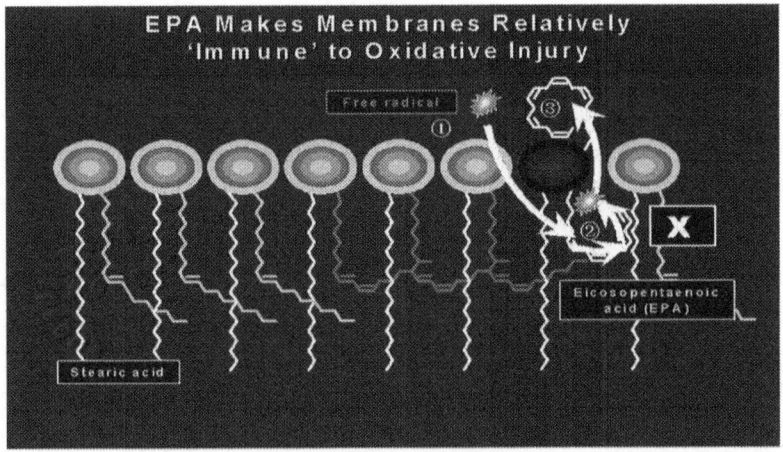

Image 25: EPA Makes Membranes Relatively
'Immune' to Oxidative Injury

Studies showing health benefits from ω-3 PUFAs have used marine-derived docosahexanenoic acid (DHA) and eicosapentaenoic acid (EPA) but <u>NOT</u> vegetable-derived α-linolenic acid (ALA). The best source of DHA/EPA is Antarctic krill, a shrimp-like crustacean consumed by whales. DHA and EPA reduce small LDL particle production (decreasing TG and increasing HDL-C). They also block oxidation (see Image 25 above) and inflammation within the body. ALA is not active in this regard and must be converted by the body into EPA to have any effect. Only a very small amount of ALA is ever converted into EPA and this conversion only decreases as we age. In the GISSI trial (Stone, Neil J et al. *Current Cardiology Reports.* 2000:2;445-451), individuals with a history of CHD who took around 850 mg of DHA plus EPA (in the form of a fish oil supplement pill—equivalent to prescription Omacor) had 41% fewer future CV events compared to similar individuals who took a placebo pill. Therefore, focus on marine sources of DHA and EPA rather than vegetable sources of ALA (canola oil, walnuts, flaxseed, flaxseed oil) to get <u>AT LEAST</u> 1000 mg of ω-3 PUFAs each day (see Table 5 below).

Source	Serving Size for 1000 mg DHA+EPA
Bass, fresh-water	4.6 oz
Bass, striped	3.7 oz
Bluefish	3.6 oz
Calamari	7.2 oz
Catfish, channel, wild	14.9 oz
Cod, Atlantic	22.3 oz
Dolphinfish	25.5 oz
Flounder (or Sole)	7.1 oz
Grouper	14.2 oz
Haddock	14.9 oz
Halibut	7.6 oz
Herring, Atlantic	1.8 oz
Lobster, northern	42.1 oz
Mackerel, Atlantic	2.9 oz
Mullet	10.8 oz
Perch, ocean	9.2 oz
Pompano	4.8 oz
Rockfish	8.0 oz
Roughy, orange	114 oz
Salmon, Atlantic, farmed	1.3 oz
Salmon, Atlantic, wild	1.9 oz
Salmon, coho, farmed	2.8 oz
Salmon, coho, wild	3.3 oz
Scallops	9.7 oz
Sea Bass	4.6 oz
Shark	4.2 oz
Shrimp	11.2 oz
Snapper	11.0 oz
Swordfish	4.3 oz

Source	Serving Size for 1000 mg DHA+EPA
Tilapia	26.1 oz
Tilefish	3.9 oz
Trout, rainbow, farmed	3.1 oz
Trout, rainbow, wild	3.6 oz
Tuna, bluefin	2.4 oz
Tuna, yellowtail	15.9 oz

Table 5. Top Food Sources of DHA+EPA

⚗

Omega-9 Fats are Good

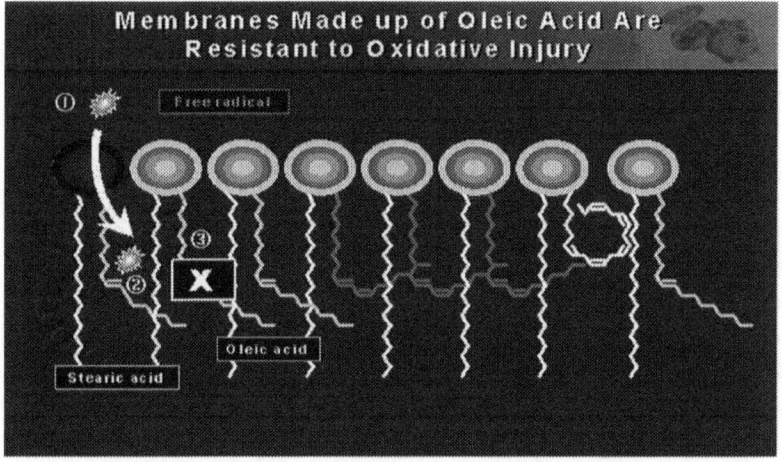

Image 26: Membranes Made up of Oleic Acid Are
Resistant to Oxidative Injury

Omega-9 monounsaturated fatty acids (ω-9 MUFAs) can decrease production of both large as well as small LDL particles (decreasing LDL-C and increasing HDL-C). They also make the body more resistant to oxidation (see Image 26 above) and inflammation. The most common ω-9 MUFA is oleic acid. Omega-9 MUFAs are found in highest concentration in dietary oils (such as olive oil), nuts (especially macadamia nuts), fish (especially swordfish), meats (especially lean cuts of beef) and some other foods (like avocadoes). You should get 20–40% of your total daily calories from ω-9 MUFAs on the HAPI Heart Diet.

Final Word on Fats—Heroes & Villains

Now let's examine various fat-containing foods (non-fish meats, fish/shellfish, dietary oils and nuts/seeds) in regards to their composition of 'good' versus 'bad' fats and see how we can use this information to determine which foods should be avoided and which foods should be consumed in states of excessive large and/or small LDL particles. People with CV disease, type II DM, high risk for future CV disease and/or obesity should follow the small LDL particle charts. Oleic acid is represented by ω-9 MUFA, linoleic acid by ω-6 PUFA and DHA+EPA by ω-3 PUFA.

Non-Fish Meat	Chol (mg)	SFA (g)	ω-9 MUFA (g)	ω-3 PUFA (g)	ω-6 PUFA (g)	ω-9:6 ratio	ω-3:6 ratio
Bacon (pork) 2 slices	18	2.10	2.59	0	0.618	4.2	0
Beef (tenderloin) 4 oz	89	3.38	3.28	0	0.259	12.7	0
Bison (sirloin) 4 oz	97	2.73	2.29	0	0.232	9.9	0
Chicken (breast) 4 oz	96	1.14	1.18	0	0.667	1.77	0
Duck (breast) 4 oz	162	0.65	0.90	0	0.341	2.64	0

Non-Fish Meat	Chol (mg)	SFA (g)	ω-9 MUFA (g)	ω-3 PUFA (g)	ω-6 PUFA (g)	ω-9:6 ratio	ω-3:6 ratio
Egg (chicken) 1 large	212	1.63	1.86	0	0.594	3.13	0
Frankfurter (beef) 1 unit	24	5.26	5.59	0	0.453	12.3	0
Hamburger (lean) 1 patty	62	2.44	2.13	0	0.197	10.8	0
Lamb (shank) 4 oz	119	6.31	5.78	0	0.818	7.07	0
Pork (tenderloin) 4 oz	89	1.88	1.94	0	0.395	4.91	0
Sausage (pork) 2 links	18	3.37	4.11	0	0.900	4.57	0
Turkey (breast) 4 oz	94	0.27	0.124	0	0.147	0.84	0
Veal (sirloin) 4 oz	118	2.72	2.23	0	0.407	5.48	0
Venison (tenderloin) 4 oz	99	1.29	0.499	0	0.085	5.87	0

Table 6. Fats in Non-Fish Meats

Non-Fish Meat	
Turkey (breast)	Best Selection
Chicken (breast)	
Duck (breast)	
Venison (tenderloin)	
Pork (tenderloin)	
Egg (chicken)	
Bacon (pork)	
Hamburger (beef)	
Bison (sirloin)	
Sausage (pork)	
Beef (tenderloin)	
Veal (sirloin)	
Frankfurter (beef)	
Lamb (shank)	Worst Selection

Table 7. Selection of Non-Fish Meats for Individual with
Increased Number of Large LDL Particles

Non-Fish Meat	
Venison (tenderloin)	Best Selection
Hamburger (beef)	
Beef (tenderloin)	
Bison (sirloin)	
Pork (tenderloin)	
Chicken (breast)	
Duck (breast)	
Frankfurter (beef)	
Turkey (breast)	
Bacon (pork)	
Egg (chicken)	

Non-Fish Meat	
Sausage (pork)	
Veal (sirloin)	
Lamb (shank)	Worst Selection

Table 8. Selection of Non-Fish Meats for Individual with Increased Number of Small LDL Particles

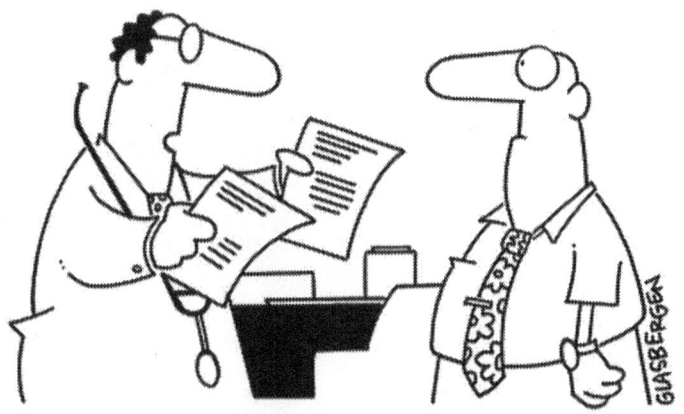

Copyright 2003 by Randy Glasbergen.
www.glasbergen.com

"On this diet, you can eat all the steak you want, but a slice of bread will kill you. On this other diet, you can eat all the bread you want, but a steak will kill you."

All the above meats are of the leanest cuts, trimmed of any visible fat (or skin in the case of poultry) and either broiled or roasted. Please realize that the consumption of any non-fish meat has repeatedly been shown to be related to increased likelihood of CV disease (as well as various malignancies). For example, the Californian Seventh Day Adventist Meat vs Vegetarian Study (Snowdon, David et al. *Preventive Medicine.* 1984:13;490-500) showed that males 45 to 54 years of age were 4.41

times more likely to die from CV disease if they consumed legged animal (non-fish) meat one to two times per week and 5.89 times more likely if they consumed such meat six or more days per week. Excessive consumption of any meat can also lead to small LDL particles (due to production of homocysteine—an amino acid metabolite that enhances tissue oxidation).

Fish and Shellfish	Chol (mg)	SFA (g)	ω-9 MUFA (g)	ω-3 PUFA (g)	ω-6 PUFA (g)	ω-9:6 ratio	ω-3:6 ratio
Bass, fresh-water 4 oz	98	1.13	1.44	0.863	0.127	11.3	6.80
Bass, striped 4 oz	116	0.73	0.65	1.092	0.021	31.0	52
Bluefish 4 oz	86	1.32	0.990	1.116	0.087	11.4	12.8
Calamari 3 oz	198	0.30	0.039	0.415	0.002	19.5	208
Catfish, channel, wild 4 oz	81	0.84	0.872	0.268	0.160	5.5	1.68
Cod, Atlantic 4 oz	62	0.19	0.088	0.179	0.007	12.6	25.6
Crab, King 1 leg	71	0.18	0.119	0.553	0.027	4.41	20.5
Dolphinfish 4 oz	106	0.27	0.124	0.157	0.052	2.38	3.02
Flounder (or Sole) 4 oz	77	0.41	0.174	0.567	0.016	10.9	35.4
Grouper 4 oz	53	0.34	0.097	0.281	0.020	4.85	14.1
Haddock 4 oz	84	0.19	0.097	0.268	0.014	6.9	19.1
Halibut 4 oz	46	0.47	0.523	0.526	0.043	12.2	12.2
Herring 4 oz	87	2.96	2.197	2.276	0.189	11.6	12.0

Fish and Shellfish	Chol (mg)	SFA (g)	ω-9 MUFA (g)	ω-3 PUFA (g)	ω-6 PUFA (g)	ω-9:6 ratio	ω-3:6 ratio
Lobster, northern 4 oz	81	0.12	0.107	0.095	0.006	17.8	15.8
Mackerel, Atlantic 4 oz	85	4.72	1.358	1.360	0.166	8.18	8.19
Mullet 4 oz	71	1.62	0.221	0.370	0.106	2.08	3.49
Perch, ocean 4 oz	61	0.35	0.299	0.432	0.041	7.29	10.5
Pompano 4 oz	72	5.08	2.930	0.823	0.175	16.7	4.70
Rockfish 4 oz	50	0.54	0.318	0.501	0.043	7.40	11.7
Roughy, orange 4 oz	90	0.04	0.331	0.035	0.064	5.17	0.55
Salmon, Atlantic, farmed 4 oz	71	2.83	2.312	3.084	0.753	3.07	4.10
Salmon, Atlantic, wild 4 oz	80	1.42	1.957	2.079	0.249	7.86	8.3
Salmon, coho, farmed 4 oz	71	2.20	2.084	1.445	0.421	4.95	3.43
Salmon, coho, wild 4 oz	62	1.19	1.787	1.197	0.063	28.4	19
Scallops 4 oz	60	0.17	0.035	0.413	0.008	4.38	51.6
Sea Bass 4 oz	60	0.74	0.426	0.861	0.035	12.2	24.6
Shark 4 oz	58	1.05	1.106	0.953	0.086	12.9	11.1
Shrimp 4 oz	220	0.33	0.129	0.356	0.024	5.38	14.8
Snapper 4 oz	53	0.41	0.139	0.362	0.028	4.96	12.9
Swordfish 4 oz	56	1.59	1.573	0.926	0.042	37.5	22.0

Fish and Shellfish	Chol (mg)	SFA (g)	ω-9 MUFA (g)	ω-3 PUFA (g)	ω-6 PUFA (g)	ω-9:6 ratio	ω-3:6 ratio
Tilapia 4 oz	64	1.06	0.864	0.153	0.322	2.68	0.48
Tilefish 4 oz	72	0.98	1.067	1.022	0.054	19.8	18.9
Trout, rainbow, farmed 4 oz	77	2.38	1.613	1.304	1.072	1.50	1.22
Trout, rainbow, wild 4 oz	78	1.83	1.037	1.117	0.325	3.19	3.44
Tuna, bluefin 4 oz	55	1.82	1.339	1.699	0.077	17.4	22.1
Tuna, yellow-tail 4 oz	66	0.34	0.156	0.315	0.011	14.2	28.6

Table 9. Fats in Fish and Shellfish

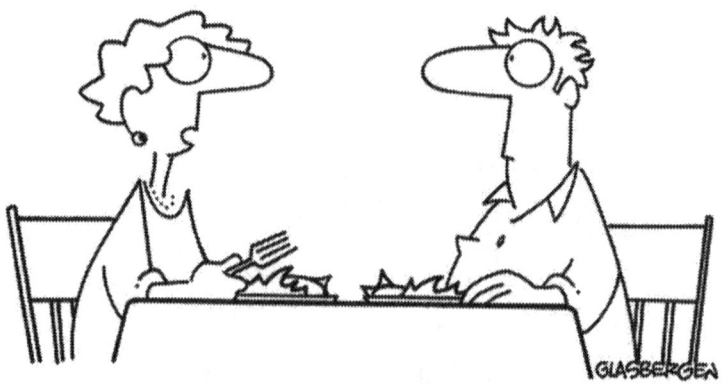

Copyright 2004 by Randy Glasbergen.
www.glasbergen.com

"If fish is the best diet food,
how come our cat weighs a ton?"

Fish and Shellfish	
Scallops	Best Selection
Grouper	
Cod, Atlantic	
Rockfish	
Snapper	
Crab, King	
Halibut	
Perch, ocean	
Tuna, yellowtail	
Lobster, northern	
Sea Bass *	
Shark *	
Roughy, orange	
Haddock	
Flounder (or Sole)	
Swordfish *	
Tilapia	
Tuna, Bluefin *	
Salmon, coho, wild *	
Dolphinfish	
Tilefish *	
Calamari	
Catfish, channel, wild	
Shrimp	
Mullet	
Bass, striped *	
Salmon, coho, farmed *	
Salmon, Atlantic, wild *	
Salmon, Atlantic, farmed *	
Trout, rainbow, wild *	
Bluefish *	
Trout, rainbow, farmed *	

Fish and Shellfish	
Bass, freshwater *	
Herring, Atlantic *	
Mackerel, Atlantic *	
Pompano *	Worst Selection

Table 10. Selection of Fish and Shellfish for Individual with Increased Number of Large LDL Particles

Fish and Shellfish	
Cod, Atlantic	Best Selection
Tuna, yellowtail	
Scallops	
Swordfish *	
Lobster, northern	
Sea Bass *	
Calamari	
Halibut	
Tuna, Bluefin *	
Salmon, coho, wild *	
Bass, striped *	
Flounder (or Sole)	
Tilefish	
Crab, King	
Grouper	
Rockfish	
Shark *	
Perch, ocean	
Haddock	
Shrimp	
Snapper	

Fish and Shellfish	
Bluefish *	
Pompano *	
Roughy, orange	
Salmon, Atlantic, wild *	
Bass, fresh-water *	
Herring, Atlantic *	
Mackerel, Atlantic *	
Catfish, channel, wild	
Tilapia	
Dolphinfish	
Salmon, coho, farmed *	
Mullet	
Salmon, Atlantic, farmed *	
Trout, rainbow, wild *	
Trout, rainbow, farmed *	Worst Selection

Table 11. Selection of Fish and Shellfish for Individual with Increased Number of Small LDL Particles

All the above fish and shellfish are fresh and cooked with either dry or moist heat. Fish marked with an asterisk (*) contain one gram or more of DHA+EPA per 4–6 oz serving. Remember that multiple scientific studies have shown that frequent consumption of almost any fish and/ or shellfish decreases the incidence of heart attack, stroke, premature CV death, type II DM as well as lethal heart rhythms. Don't eat TOO MUCH fish or shellfish since excessive meat intake can increase small LDL particle levels as described above. I would also recommend avoiding 'farm-raised' fish since they are fed soybeans and/or other similar vegetable-derived products intended for poultry and, in effect, become 'chicken with gills.'

Dietary Oil (1 T. of each)	Chol (mg)	SFA (g)	ω-9 MUFA (g)	ω-3 PUFA (g)	ω-6 PUFA (g)	ω-9:6 ratio	ω-3:6 ratio
Almond oil	0	1.12	9.438	0	2.366	3.99	0
Avocado oil	0	1.62	9.504	0	1.754	5.44	0
Butter, no salt	31	7.29	2.41-c 0.42-t	0	0.387	6.23	0
Canola oil	0	0.99	7.854	0	2.842	2.77	0
Coconut oil	0	11.8	0.789	0	0.245	3.22	0
Cod liver oil	78	3.08	2.809	2.43	0.127	22.1	19.1
Corn oil	0	1.76	3.717	0	7.278	0.51	0
Flaxseed oil	0	1.28	2.747	0	1.727	1.59	0
Grapeseed oil	0	1.31	2.149	0	9.466	0.23	0
Hazelnut oil	0	1.00	10.581	0	1.374	7.70	0
Herring oil	104	2.90	1.626	1.425	0.156	10.4	9.13
Macadamia nut oil	0	2.02	11.56	0	0.408	28.3	0
Margarine, soft	0	1.44	1.90-c 0.99-t	0	3.091	0.61	0
Olive oil	0	1.86	9.621	0	1.318	7.30	0
Palm oil	0	6.71	4.978	0	1.238	4.02	0
Palm kernel oil	0	11.1	1.550	0	0.218	7.11	0
Peanut oil	0	2.28	6.048	0	4.320	1.4	0
Safflower oil	0	0.84	1.952	0	10.149	0.19	0
Salmon oil	66	2.70	2.309	4.251	0.210	11.0	20.2
Sardine oil	97	4.07	2.006	2.828	0.274	7.32	10.3
Sesame oil	0	1.93	5.345	0	5.617	0.95	0
Soybean oil	0	1.96	3.101	0	6.936	0.45	0
Sunflower oil	0	1.40	2.652	0	8.935	0.30	0
Walnut oil	0	1.24	3.019	0	7.194	0.42	0

Table 12. Fats in Dietary Oils

Copyright 2004 by Randy Glasbergen.
www.glasbergen.com

"**Large doses of fish oil are good for your cardiovascular system. Especially if you get the urge to swim upstream.**"

<u>Dietary Oil</u>	
Safflower oil	Best Selection
Canola oil	
Hazelnut oil	
Almond oil	
Walnut oil	
Flaxseed oil	
Grapeseed oil	
Sunflower oil	
Avocado oil	
Corn oil	
Olive oil	
Sesame oil	
Soybean oil	
Macadamia nut oil	
Peanut oil	
Salmon oil	

Dietary Oil	
Herring oil	
Margarine, soft	
Cod Liver oil	
Sardine oil	
Palm oil	
Palm kernel oil	
Butter, no salt	
Coconut oil	Worst Selection

Table 13. Selection of Dietary Oil for Individual with Increased Number of Large LDL Particles

Dietary Oil	
Hazelnut oil	Best Selection
Almond oil	
Canola oil	
Macadamia nut oil	
Olive oil	
Salmon oil	
Avocado oil	
Cod liver oil	
Herring oil	
Flaxseed oil	
Safflower oil	
Sardine oil	
Walnut oil	
Corn oil	
Sesame oil	
Grapeseed oil	
Palm kernel oil	

Dietary Oil	
Sunflower oil	
Peanut oil	
Butter, no salt	
Palm oil	
Soybean oil	
Margarine, soft	
Coconut oil	Worst Selection

Table 14. Selection of Dietary Oil for Individual with Increased Number of Small LDL Particles

Nut/Seed (1 oz of each)	Chol (mg)	SFA (g)	ω-9 MUFA (g)	ω-3 PUFA (g)	ω-6 PUFA (g)	ω-9:6 ratio	ω-3:6 ratio
Almonds, raw	0	1.1	9.05	0	3.463	2.61	0
Brazilnuts, dried	0	4.3	6.87	0	5.824	1.18	0
Cashews, raw	0	2.2	6.67	0	2.206	3.02	0
Flaxseed, ground—1 T.	0	0.3	0.52	0	0.413	1.26	0
Hazelnuts, raw	0	1.3	12.87	0	2.221	5.79	0
Macadamia nuts, raw	0	3.4	12.4	0	0.367	33.8	0
Peanuts, raw	0	1.9	6.74	0	4.410	1.53	0
Pecans, raw	0	1.8	11.51	0	5.848	1.97	0
Pine nuts, dried	0	1.4	5.09	0	9.398	0.54	0
Pistachios, raw	0	1.5	6.43	0	3.742	1.72	0
Pumpkin seeds, dried	0	2.5	4.01	0	5.869	0.70	0
Sunflower seeds, dried	0	1.5	2.65	0	9.251	0.29	0

Nut/Seed (1 oz of each)	Chol (mg)	SFA (g)	ω-9 MUFA (g)	ω-3 PUFA (g)	ω-6 PUFA (g)	ω-9:6 ratio	ω-3:6 ratio
Walnuts, raw	0	1.7	2.50	0	10.80	0.23	0

Table 15. Fats in Nuts & Seeds

Nut/Seed	
Flaxseed, ground	Best Selection
Almonds, raw	
Hazelnuts, raw	
Pine nuts, dried	
Pistachios, raw	
Sunflower seeds, dried	
Walnuts, raw	
Pecans, raw	
Peanuts, raw	
Cashews, raw	
Pumpkin seeds, dried	
Macadamia nuts, raw	
Brazilnuts, dried	Worst Selection

Table 15. Selection of Nuts & Seeds for Individual with Increased Number of Large LDL Particles

Nut/Seed	
Hazelnuts, raw	Best Selection
Almonds, raw	
Macadamia nuts, raw	
Flaxseed, ground	

Nut/Seed	
Cashews, raw	
Pistachios, raw	
Pecans, raw	
Peanuts, raw	
Pine nuts, dried	
Sunflower seeds, dried	
Brazilnuts, dried	
Pumpkin seeds, dried	
Walnuts, raw	Worst Selection

Table 16. Selection of Nuts & Seeds for Individual with Increased Number of Small LDL Particles

Part II. Carbohydrates

Carbohydrates should constitute about 20–40% of your total daily calories on the HAPI Heart Diet. Carbohydrates contain four calories per gram. Carbohydrates are found in a wide variety of foods and are one of the three major macronutrients that supply the body with energy (fat and protein being the others). But, unlike fat and protein, carbohydrates are efficiently converted into glucose, which is directly used by the muscles and brain. In fact, the Institute of Medicine (IOM) has recommended that all children and adults get a minimum of 130 grams of carbohydrate per day to maintain maximal brain function. Carbohydrates play an important role in the construction and maintenance of the body's tissues, organs and cells. For optimal health, consume a wide range of carbohydrate-containing food such as whole grains, fresh fruits and vegetables as well as low-fat dairy products. These foods provide a variety of other important substances, such as vitamins, minerals, phytochemicals and antioxidants. Each of your four to six main meals per day should contain a balanced amount of carbohydrate in relationship to fat and protein. Your post-workout meal(s) should contain 60–75% high-GI carbohydrate (see below) and 25–40% protein.

Whole grains should be listed first on the ingredient list of any food label. Examples of whole grains include whole wheat flour, oatmeal, corn, popcorn, whole cornmeal, brown rice, graham flour, whole rye flour, barley and wild rice. Whole grains contain the entire grain kernel—the bran (rich in fiber), the germ (rich in vitamins and minerals) and the endosperm (the starchy part). Note that 'wheat flour' is not a whole grain; the label must say 'whole wheat flour' to count as a whole grain.

Carbohydrates can be broken down into fiber, sugars and starches. Starches are converted into sugars with the amount of fiber slowing down this process by delaying the absorption and breakdown of starches (as well as sugars). Commonly called roughage, fiber is an indigestible complex carbohydrate found in plants that has no calories because the body cannot absorb it. Fiber helps decrease the production and enhance the clearance of large LDL particles.

Fiber can be broken down into soluble fiber and insoluble (or viscous) fiber. Sources of soluble fiber include the skins of fruits (apples, pears, peaches, grapes), the piths of oranges, the skins of vegetables, seeds, nuts, pectin, oat bran, psyllium, dried beans, oatmeal, guar, barley, rye and prunes. Sources of insoluble fiber include the 'meat' of fruits and vegetables, dried beans, wheat bran, seeds, nuts, brown rice, popcorn as well as whole-grain breads, cereals and pastas. Thus the main sources of fiber are fruits, seeds, nuts, vegetables and whole grains.

Besides improving bowel function, fiber has been found to reduce the risk of CHD (by 40 percent in some studies), type II DM, diverticular disease and possibly colon cancer. Certain fibers (called cellulose and hemicellulose) also take up space in the gastrointestinal tract without yielding any calories, promoting a feeling of fullness.

You should get at least 25 to 35 grams of supplemental fiber every day on the HAPI Heart Diet. Fiber supplements can be taken with your main meals for this purpose (I personally take two Fiber Choice sugar-free wafers each containing four grams of soluble fiber with every main meal). Remember to add fiber gradually to your diet to prevent bloating, gas, diarrhea and abdominal discomfort.

Δ
Glycemic Index

The glycemic index (GI) measures how fast a food (carbohydrate) is likely to raise your blood sugar and blood insulin levels (see Table 5 below). For example, if your blood sugar drops during exercise, consume a carbohydrate with a higher GI ($\geq$ 70; thus more quickly absorbed). On the other hand, if you want to keep your blood sugar from dropping during a few hours of mild activity, consume a carbohydrate that has a lower GI ($\leq$ 55; thus more slowly absorbed). Therefore, if your blood sugar spikes after breakfast, select a cereal with a lower GI.

The GI of any particular food is determined relative to that of glucose, which is given an arbitrary value of 100. Basically, the more sugar/starch any particular carbohydrate has relative to fiber, the higher its GI will be and the more fiber any particular carbohydrate has relative to sugar/starch, the lower its GI will be. Thus, one way to lower the 'relative' GI of any particular food/carbohydrate is to take it with a fiber supplement.

	GI		GI
BAKERY GOODS		Pineapple juice, unsweetened	46
Angel food cake	67	Tomato juice, canned	38
Banana cake	47	Gatorade	78
Chocolate cake	38	Quik, chocolate	41
Cupcake	73	Quik, strawberry	35

	GI		GI
Pound cake	54	BREADS	
Sponge cake	46	Bagel	72
Vanilla cake	42	Baguette	95
Croissant	67	Hamburger bun	61
Doughnut	76	Kaiser roll	73
Apple muffin	44	Melba toast	70
Banana muffin	65	Oat bran bread	47
Bran muffin	60	Pumpernickel bread	55
Blueberry muffin	59	Rye bread	58
Carrot muffin	62	Sourdough bread	53
Corn muffin	102	Whole wheat bread	52
Oatmeal	69	White bread	70
Pancakes	67	Wonder, white bread	73
Scones	92	Semolina bread	64
Waffles	76	Middle Eastern flatbread	97
BEVERAGES		Pita bread	57
Coca Cola	63	CEREALS	
Smoothie	33	All-Bran	42
Apple juice, unsweetened	40	Bran Buds	58
Carrot juice	43	Bran Flakes	74
Cranberry juice cocktail	68	Cheerios	74
Grapefruit juice, unsweetened	48	Coco Pops	77
Orange juice, unsweetened	53	Corn Chex	83
CEREALS		Rice, Basmati, white	58
Cornflakes	81	Rice, brown	55
Corn Pops	80	Rice, parboiled	72
Cream of Wheat	66	Rye, whole kernels	34
Froot Loops	69	Wheat, whole kernels	41
Frosted Flakes	55	Semolina	55

	GI		GI
Golden Grahams	71	Bulgur	48
Grapenuts	71	COOKIES	
Grapenuts Flakes	80	Oatmeal	54
Honey Smacks	71	Shortbread	64
Just Right	60	Vanilla Wafers	77
Life	66	CRACKERS	
Muesli	66	Puffed rice cakes	78
Nutrigrain	66	Stoned Wheat Thins	67
Oat bran, raw	55	Soda Crackers	74
Raisin Bran	61	MILK PRODUCTS	
Rice Krispies	82	Custard	38
Shredded Wheat	75	Ice cream, chocolate	37
Special K	69	Ice cream, French vanilla	38
Total	76	Milk, full-fat	27
GRAINS		Milk, skim	32
Barley	25	Milk, condensed	61
Buckwheat	54	Mousse	34
Cornmeal	69	Pudding	44
Taco shells	68	Yogurt, low-fat, fruit	33
Couscous	65	Soy milk, full-fat	44
Rice, Arborio (risotto)	69	Soy milk, reduced-fat	44
Rice, white, long grain	56	Tofu frozen dessert	115
Rice, Jasmine, long grain	109		
FRUITS		Navy beans	38
Apples, raw	38	Kidney beans	28
Apricots, raw	57	Black beans	20
Cantaloupe, raw	65	Lentils, green	30
Banana, raw	52	Lentils, red	26
Cherries, raw	22	Lima beans	32
Dates, dried	103	Peas	22
Figs, dried	61	Pinto beans	42
Fruit Cocktail	55	Split peas, yellow	32

	GI		GI
Grapefruit, raw	25	PASTAS	
Grapes, raw	46	Capellini	45
Kiwi fruit, raw	53	Fettucine	40
Lychee, canned	79	Gnocchi	68
Mango, raw	51	Linguine	46
Oranges, raw	42	Angel hair	52
Papaya, raw	59	Macaroni	47
Peach, raw	42	Macaroni and Cheese	64
Pear, raw	38	Spaghetti, protein enriched	27
Pineapple, raw	59	Spaghetti, white, boiled 5 min	38
Plum, raw, NS	39	Spaghetti, white, boiled 15 min	44
Prunes, pitted	29	Tortellini, cheese	50
Raisins	64	Vermicelli	35
Strawberries, raw	40	SNACKS	
Watermelon, raw	72	Corn chips	63
LEGUMES		Fruit Roll-Ups	99
Baked beans	40	Jelly beans	78
Black-eyed peas	42	Kudos Bars	62
Butter beans	31	Life Savers	70
Chickpeas	28	M & M's, peanut	33
SNACKS		VEGETABLES	
Mars Bar	65	Broad beans	79
Nutella	33	Green peas	48
Cashew nuts	22	Pumpkin	75
Peanuts	14	Sweet corn, on the cob	48
Popcorn	72	Sweet corn, fresh	54
Pop Tarts	70	Sweet corn, canned	46
Pretzels, wheat	83	Sweet corn, frozen	47
Skittles	70	Carrots, raw	16
Snickers Bar	55	Cassava	46
Twix Bar	44	Parsnips	97
Power Bar	56	Potato, baked	85

	GI		GI
<u>SOUPS</u>		French Fries	75
Black Bean	64	Potato, mashed	74
Green Pea	66	Potato, new	57
Lentil	44	Sweet potato	61
Minestrone	39	Tapioca	81
Split Pea	60	Taro	55
Tomato	38	Yam	37

<u>Table 5. Glycemic Index (GI) of Many Common Foods</u>

The impact a food will have on blood sugar depends on other factors such as ripeness, cooking time, protein and fat content, time of day and recent physical activity. One quick and super-simple way to get the same sort of information as the GI is to take the total grams of carbohydrate for one serving of a particular food and subtract the total grams of fiber the serving contains from that number.

Many hormones are involved with determining the body's BMR. One of the most influential of these is insulin. Insulin is a hormone secreted by the pancreas as a response to elevated blood sugar levels that serves to move that 'excess' sugar out of the bloodstream and into the appropriate tissues of the body (i.e. liver, muscles, fat reserves). Under normal physiologic, nutritional and behavioral conditions, blood insulin and corresponding blood sugar levels are relatively low and 'under control.'

Many people can develop problems with what is termed 'insulin resistance' (IR)—which means that the tissues of their bodies do not respond adequately (in the uptake of excess blood sugar) to normal blood insulin levels and this thereby leads to 'hyperinsulinemia' or elevated blood insulin levels.

Elevated blood insulin levels slow down the body's BMR by several major mechanisms: 1) increasing hunger with cravings mainly for refined carbohydrates (sugars and starches) which lead to further blood insulin 'spikes' when those carbohydrates are quickly digested; 2) making you feel sleepier, less likely to exercise and more likely to take a nap (your BMR is quite low while you are sleeping); & 3) increasing those fat reserves that surround the intestinal structures (leading to the classic 'beer gut') which makes the tissues of the body even that much more resistant to insulin.

This cycle of IR leading to hyperinsulinemia leading to further IR eventually leads to obesity and sometimes even to type II DM. The current thought is that 90% of type II DM is caused by obesity, lack of sufficient daily physical activity and daily over-consumption of refined carbohydrates. Excessive intake of high-GI carbohydrates increases hepatic TG production and resultant elevated blood insulin levels increase small LDL particle concentrations as well as tissue oxidation and inflammation.

An extremely powerful trick in modifying your BMR to enhance weight loss is to avoid the consumption of high-GI carbohydrates and other substances (salt/sodium as well as artificial sweeteners) that lead to elevations of blood insulin levels. Understand that the lower your daily consumption of sugar, starch, salt/sodium and artificial sweeteners, the lower your insulin level, the more regulated your blood sugar level, the higher your energy level, the lower your hunger and the smaller (eventually) your waistline. Remember, the more high-GI carbohydrates you eat, the more you want to eat; the less high-GI carbohydrates you eat, the less you care to eat.

Copyright 2003 by Randy Glasbergen.
www.glasbergen.com

**"I'm on a low-carb diet.
Whenever I feel low, I eat carbs!"**

Part III. Protein

Protein should constitute 20–30% of your total daily calories on the HAPI Heart Diet. Protein contains four calories per gram. Protein is the fundamental structural material of all cells of the body as well as biologically active substances such as cell membrane receptors, enzymes, hormones, immunoglobulins, neuotransmitters as well as storage and transport compounds. The building blocks of all human proteins are 20 amino acids that may be consumed from both animal and plant sources. Of these 20 amino acids, nine are considered 'essential' since they can not be created by the body and must therefore be present in the diet (see Table 4 below). Protein from animal sources (meat including fish and shellfish, dairy products, egg white) is considered 'complete' because all nine essential amino acids are present whereas protein from plant sources (grains, legumes, nuts and seeds) is usually considered 'incomplete' since several of the essential amino acids may be absent.

Essential Amino Acids	Nonessential Amino Acids
Histidine	Alanine
Isoleucine	Arginine

Essential Amino Acids	Nonessential Amino Acids
Leucine	Aspartic acid
Lysine	Cysteine
Methionine	Cystine
Phenylalanine	Glutamic acid
Threonine	Glutamine
Tryptophan	Glycine
Valine	Proline
	Serine
	Tyrosine

Table 6. Essential vs Nonessential Amino Acids

Each main meal should contain a balanced amount of protein in relationship to fat and carbohydrate. Post-workout meals should contain 25–40% protein and 60–75% high-GI carbohydrate. Excessive protein intake can elevate blood insulin levels, increase small LDL particle levels as well as enhance tissue oxidation and inflammation (due to increased blood homocysteine levels). Please recall that a low-fat, low-carbohydrate, high-protein liquid diet was used in the relatively recent past to promote weight loss and worked quite well for this but also ended up killing a number of individuals from lethal heart rhythms.

Part IV. Water

You should drink at least six to eight 8-oz glasses of water each day on the HAPI Heart Diet. Water is required for almost all chemical reactions involved in body metabolism, so if you are dehydrated, your BMR may slow down as a response in order to return to a state of homeostasis. Remember to drink your water right before or in between meals and not WITH meals. Drinking a lot of water while you are consuming your food may dilute your digestive enzymes and impede your digestion. Your body may respond to this by decreasing BMR. On the contrary, drinking green, red or white tea or a small amount of alcohol along with meals assists digestion and may enhance BMR. Consumption of green, red or white tea can decrease large LDL particle levels while (in most people) modest alcohol intake (one drink per day for women and one to two drinks per day for men) can help decrease small LDL particle levels. Note that excessive alcohol consumption usually increases small LDL particle levels. One cup of filtered, caffeinated coffee per day (or one 'shot' of espresso) is probably fine but more than this actually tends to decrease BMR over time.

Since a lot of hunger is actually thirst in disguise in our 'modern' world where we basically exist in the semi-dehydrated state (consuming a lot of salt and/or sugar, drinking alcohol, cola, coffee and/or tea which all dehydrate the body—becoming prunes instead of plums and raisins instead of grapes), drinking a large amount of water each and every day will also help lower your desire for food. Foodstuffs obviously contain water so many times our cravings for food are actually cravings for water being misinterpreted. You can prove this to yourself: sit down at the table with a plate of something you typically crave (e.g. pizza). Get a sense of your desire for the pizza and then drink an 8-oz glass of water. You will note your cravings soon diminish. Do it the next time with a can of soda (full of sugar); you'll note your cravings soon intensify due to increased blood insulin.

Part V. Sodium

You should consume less than two grams of salt/sodium each day on the HAPI Heart Diet. Excessive sodium intake can lead to fluid retention, elevations in blood pressure, increased stress upon the CV system, increased hunger, tissue oxidation and inflammation, diminished rate of metabolism as well as increased small LDL particle concentrations. Some tricks to lower your sodium intake include: 1) don't <u>EVER</u> use the salt shaker; 2) don't eat foods where you can actually see salt crystals or taste the salt just by licking (crackers, pretzels, nuts, chips); 3) avoid cheeses, canned soups and canned vegetables; 4) minimize bakery products (breads, cakes, pasta, noodles, rolls, cookies); 5) avoid salted meats (bacon, ham); and 6) avoid going out to eat but, if you must, make a big deal to the server and/or chef—"Please, please, PLEASE, no salt." Remember that the vast majority of salt (probably around 90%) consumed by the 'average' American comes from packaged, processed foods as well as going out to eat and not from the salt shaker.

Part VI. Vitamins and Minerals

Vitamins are organic compounds that assist with various biologic processes to release energy from digested foodstuffs and thus are essential to life. Since the body is unable to synthesize vitamins, they must be ingested to maintain adequate levels within the body. Together with minerals, they are considered 'micro'-nutrients since the body requires them in much smaller quantities than it does 'macro'-nutrients such as carbohydrates, fats, protein and water. Since micronutrients are necessary for appropriate body functioning, if they are in short supply, BMR usually declines as a response.

In an ideal world we would get all the vitamins and minerals we require from fresh, natural foods (see Tables 5 and 6 below). However in this real world of high stress and multiple toxins, our nutritional requirements have been increasing at the very same time that our caloric needs are actually decreasing (due to diminished levels of physical activity) and much of our food is being produced devoid of many important micronutrients. According to the U.S. Department of Agriculture, around 40% of Americans regularly consume a diet consisting of just about 60% of the RDA (recommended daily allowance) of many important vitamins and minerals. Please remember that the RDA represents the average amount needed to prevent a deficiency state in the typical individual and in no way indicates the optimal amount required for any one particular person. Probably at least 50% of the U.S. population suffers from a deficiency state of at least one vital micronutrient.

Vitamin A (Retinol)
 RDA
  Men 600 mcg
  Women 600 mcg
  Children 600 mcg
  Infants 350 mcg
  Lactating Women 950 mcg
	Carrots & Sweet Potatoes
	 Parley &Spinach & Broccoli
	 Mangoes & Persimmon
	 Apricots & Oranges
	 Raspberries
	 Liver
	 Milk & Milk Products

Vitamin B1 (Thiamine)
 RDA
  Men 1.3 mg
  Women 1.0 mg
  Children 1.1 mg
  Infants 50 mcg
	Whole-Grain Cereals
	 Soya Beans
	 Turnip Greens
	 Apricots & Pineapples
	 Pistachio Nuts
	 Pork, Lamb & Liver

Vitamin B2 (Riboflavin)
 RDA
  Men 1.5 mg
  Women 1.2 mg
  Children 1.3 mg
  Infants 60 mcg
	Turnip Greens
	 Radish Leaves
	 Papayas, Apricots & Raisins
	 Liver
	 Milk & Milk Products
	 Eggs

Vitamin B3 (Niacin)
 RDA
  Men 17 mg
  Women 13 mg
  Children 15 mg
  Infants 650 mcg
	Liver
	 Pork
	 Lean Meats & Prawns
	 Milk & Milk Products
	 Rice Bran & Wheat
	 Sunflower Seeds & Almonds
	 Celery Leaves

Vitamin B5 (Pantothenic Acid)
 RDA
  Men 10 mg
  Women 10 mg
  Children 5.5 mg
	Split Peas & Soya Beans
	 Yeast
	 Liver
	 Eggs
	 Peanuts, Mushrooms

Vitamin B-6 (Pyridoxine)
 RDA
  Men 2.0 mg
  Women 2.0 mg
  Children 1.7 mg
  Infants 0.1–0.4 mg
	Bananas
	 Liver
	 Fish
	 Poultry
	 Nuts & Seeds
	 Potatoes & Sweet Potatoes
	 Whole-Grain Cereals
	 Wheat Germ & Lentils

Vitamin B8 (Biotin)	Brewer's Yeast, Wheat Germ
RDA	Liver
Men 100–200 mcg	Eggs
Women 100–200 mcg	Fatty Fish
Children 50–200 mcg	Rice Bran, Rice Germ
Infants 35 mcg	Wholemeal Bread
	Peanut Butter
	Milk & Milk Products
Vitamin B9 (Folic Acid)	Dark Green Vegetables
RDA	Spinach & Mint
Men 100 mcg	Dry Beans, Peas & Lentils
Women 100 mcg	Enriched Grain Products
Children 80 mcg	Fortified Cereals
Infants 25 mcg	Orange Juice
Pregnant Women 400 mcg	Wheat Germ & Yeast
Lactating Women 150 mcg	Liver, Meat
Vitamin B12 (Cyanocobalamin)	Eggs
RDA	Fish & Shellfish
Men 2 mcg	Fortified Cereals
Women 2 mcg	Meat
Children 1 mcg	Milk & Milk Products
Infants 0.5 mcg	Organ Meats
Lactating Women 2.6 mcg	
Vitamin C (Ascorbic Acid)	Raw Green Bell Peppers
RDA	Raw Red Bell Peppers
Men 40 mg	Brussels Sprouts
Women 40 mg	Parsley, Raw Cabbage
Children 40 mg	Tomatoes, Oranges
Infants 25 mg	Kiwi Fruit, Mangoes
Lactating Women 80 mg	Strawberries
Vitamin D	Egg Yolk
RDA	Fortified Cereals
Men 0.01 mg	Fortified Milk
Women 0.01 mg	Liver
Children 0.01 mg	High-Fat Fish

Vitamin E (Tocopherol)
RDA
  Men 15 mg
  Women 12 mg
  Children 8.3 mg
  Infants 4–5 mg
	Margarine &Vegetable Oils
	Nuts & Seeds
	Peanuts & Peanut Butter
	Wheat Germ
	Whole-Grain Cereals
	Shrimp

Vitamin K
RDA
  Men 70–140 mcg
  Women 70–140 mcg
  Children 35–75 mcg
	Broccoli & Brussels Sprouts
	Cauliflower & Cabbage
	Leafy Green Vegetables
	Mayonnaise
	Soybean, Canola & Olive Oils

Table 7. Vitamins in Food

Calcium
RDA
  Men 1200 mg
  Women 1200 mg
  Children 800 mg
  Infants 500 mg
  Pregnant Women 1200 mg
  Lactating Women 1200 mg
	Milk & Milk Products
	Cauliflower
	Carrots
	Radishes
	Coconut
	Almonds
	Fish

Chlorine
RDA
  Men 750 mg
  Women 750 mg
  Children 600 mg
	Barley, Wheat & other Grains
	Green Leafy Vegetables
	Melons
	Pineapples

Iodine
RDA
  Men 150 mcg
  Women 150 mcg
  Children 83 mcg
	Iodized Salt
	Saltwater Fish & Shellfish
	Spinach

Magnesium
RDA
  Men 350 mg
  Women 300 mg
  Children 150–200 mg
  Infants 40–60 mg
	Cocoa & Chocolate
	Dark Green Vegetables
	Dry Beans, Peas & Lentils
	Fish
	Nuts & Seeds
	Whole Grains, Brown Rice
	Apples, Figs, Lemons, Peaches

Phosphorus
RDA
  Men 1200 mg
  Women 1200 mg
  Children 800 mg
	Dry Beans, Peas & Lentils
	Eggs
	Meat, Poultry & Fish
	Milk & Milk Products
	Nuts, Seeds & Whole Grains

Potassium
RDA
  Men 2000 mg
  Women 2000 mg
  Children 1500 mg
	Legumes
	Green Leafy Vegetables
	Limes
	Peaches
	Apricots

Sodium
RDA
  Men 500 mg
  Women 500 mg
  Children 400 mg
	Green Leafy Vegetables
	Fruits
	Fish
	Meat

Zinc
RDA
  Men 15 mg
  Women 12 mg
  Children 10 mg
  Infants 5 mg
	Dry Beans, Peas & Lentils
	Meat
	Poultry
	Seeds
	Shellfish
	Whole-Grain Cereals

Table 8. Minerals in Food

In order to provide sufficient vitamins and minerals for the optimal functioning of the body, nutritional supplements may sometimes be required. One main problem with such products in this country is that the vast majority of them are in the 'dietary supplement' category without any direct FDA oversight whatsoever in terms of their safety, efficacy, quality, content or lot variability.

Although it is true that recent medical studies have failed to prove the CV benefit of various vitamin supplements, it is possible that the doses used in the studies were insufficient. For instance, if penicillin was studied in the treatment of pneumonia at a dose of just once per day (instead of the 'correct' dose of four times per day), the results of such a study would imply that penicillin was ineffective (even though we all realize this conclusion would be invalid).

On the contrary, please remember that the idea vitamins and minerals are helpful in preventing disease and promoting health comes from studies on diets rich in fresh fruit and vegetables and NOT from studies examining actual vitamin and/or mineral supplements. Obviously individuals who consume a diet rich in fresh fruit and vegetables are less likely to smoke, less likely to abuse alcohol or other drugs, more likely to exercise, more likely to be educated, more likely to enjoy a higher socioeconomic standard, more likely to seek appropriate health care and more likely to follow medical recommendations (thus more likely to 'take care of themselves' otherwise). These associated behaviors could be the main reason for the disease prevention/health promotion and not just the diet.

Even if it IS the fruits and vegetables that are directly involved, maybe there are other as of yet unidentified phytochemicals found in the actual food that are beneficial and not just the vitamins and minerals of which we know. Finally, even if it is the vitamins and minerals, maybe it's those created under 'natural' circumstances and not those manufactured synthetically. For example, vitamin E found in nature is a 'right-handed' molecule whereas vitamin E created synthetically is 50% right-handed and 50% left-handed. Who's to say that 'left-handed' vitamin E isn't actually detrimental to overall health?

Sample Patient Case #3

José is a 58 year-old overweight Hispanic-American man with type II DM, HTN and dyslipoproteiniemia. He decides to begin the HAPI Heart Diet. He determines how many calories he should consume each day based on his height and daily activity level. He will get around 40% of his daily calories from fat. He will decrease his TFA intake by avoiding butter, margarine, fast-food restaurants and processed bakery goods. He will decrease his ω-6 PUFA intake by avoiding margarine, chicken and other poultry as well as all vegetable oils except canola and olive oil. He will decrease his SFA and dietary cholesterol intake by consuming only low-fat dairy products, using Egg Beaters instead of eggs and eating small portions of lean cuts of pork or beef only once per week. José will increase his DHA+EPA (ω-3 PUFA) intake by consuming small portions of wild Coho salmon, sea bass or sword-fish almost every day. He will increase his ω-9 MUFA intake by using lots of olive oil as well as snacking on small handfuls of raw almonds, cashews, macadamia nuts and/or pecans. José will get about 30% of his calories from carbohydrates, focusing on low-GI fresh fruits and vegetables (rich in micronutrients), low-fat dairy products and small servings of wild rice or whole grain breads, cereals or pastas (rich in fiber). He will take two Fiber Choice sugar-free wafers with breakfast, lunch and dinner. He will get about 30% of his calories from protein, focusing on black and red beans, chickpeas, non-fat cottage cheese and only small portions of any kind of meat. He will drink at least eight 8-oz glasses of water per day, two in the AM upon awakening, one before breakfast, one before a mid-morning snack, one before lunch, one before a mid-afternoon snack, one before dinner and one before bedtime. He will drink 3 cups of green tea each day, one with break-fast, one with lunch and one with dinner. José will limit his sodium intake by never using the salt shaker, avoiding packaged snack foods, canned items, bakery goods and salted meats as well as only going out to eat only on special occasions.

Chapter Five
HAPI Diet Principle #3: 'Exercise More'

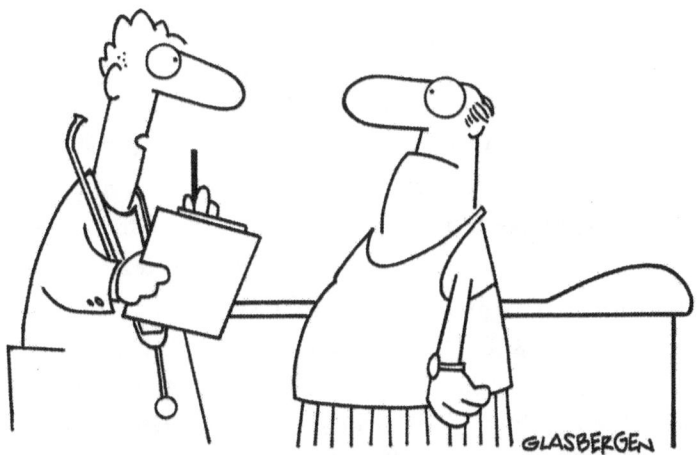

Copyright 2003 by Randy Glasbergen. www.glasbergen.com

**"What fits your busy schedule better, exercising
one hour a day or being dead 24 hours a day?"**

Burn Off More Calories Every Day

Along with decreasing your daily caloric intake, you must increase
your daily caloric expenditure, primarily by enhancing your daily physical activity (especially aerobic-based which burns off the most calories).

The goal is to build up to at least 60 minutes of exercise equivalent to the strenuousness of a brisk walk at least five or six days each and every week (see Table 12 below). You can do the exercise all at one setting or break it up into two to three segments of 20 to 30 minutes. At least 60% of the total duration of your exercise should be spent doing aerobic activity (such as walking, swimming or biking) with a goal of maintaining 60–85% of your target heart rate (THR) for the duration of the activity. THR is calculated as 220 minus your age in years. 20–30% of the total duration of your exercise should be focused on muscle strengthening (upper body one day and lower body the next) and 10–20% should be spent on stretching. Obviously you should ONLY start a daily exercise program if you are physically capable of such activity. It is VERY wise to check with your personal physician first before beginning any exercise program.

As an example of the importance of exercise, we all recognize that sumu wresters (at least the good ones) are extraordinarily overweight. But, during their careers (when they consume incredible amounts of calories but also exercise religiously), they DO NOT have small LDL particles or other signs of CV risk or MS/IR whatsoever (their excess fat is concentrated right beneath the skin surface and not in the abdominal cavity). But, as soon as their careers end and they stop exercising, things rapidly change such that fat disappears from the tissue beneath the skin and develops instead in the abdominal cavity, corresponding to elevated levels of small LDL particles, other signs of MS/IR and heightened CV risk. Think about that: when they were overweight, eating excessively but also exercising fervently, they had low CV risk; when they were equally overweight, now eating less but also exercising much less, they had high CV risk. So, exercise is dramatically helpful to decrease CV risk by itself, regardless of whether or not it leads to weight loss. Of course, doing BOTH is even better.

Once it has been determined (e.g. by your personal physician) that you are physically capable of pursuing an exercise program, please begin with the equivalent of a five to ten minute daily walk. Increase this slowly (as tolerated by your own body) by five to ten minute increments every week or so until you get to the level of the 60 minute daily walk (or whichever equivalent you prefer—swimming, biking, using the rowing machine, treadmill, stationary bike, etc...). By the way, please note the increased number of calories you tend to burn when you perform activities also involving the upper extremities. The upper extremities are much less energy efficient than the lower extremities so if you want to expend the maximal number of calories during exercise, please pursue aerobic activities using the muscle groups of your arms as well as your legs. I would avoid running or jogging since these activities cause way too much joint stress and eventual injury to the hips and knees over time. Once again, unless you want to keep the next generation of orthopedic surgeons busy, please avoid jogging and running (speed-walking is probably fine).

Activity (60 minutes)	Calories (150# person)
Aerobics	405
Backpacking	405
Badminton (singles)	684
Ballet	342
Ballroom dancing	306
Baseball	351
Basketball (1/2 court)	405
Biking (flat surface)	441
Brushing teeth	171
Climbing Stairs	612
Dancing (getting real funky)	342
Frisbee	216
Gardening	324
Golfing (no carts)	261
Grocery shopping	243
Handball	702

Activity (60 minutes)	Calories (150# person)
Hiking	414
Horseback riding	288
Housecleaning	432
Ice hockey	468
Ice skating	414
Indoor skiing (machine)	648
Ironing	153
Jogging	675
Jumping Rope	684
Karate	441
Kayaking (flat water)	405
Kissing (maybe how you do it)	72
Lacrosse	468
Mopping up after guests leave	306
Mowing the lawn (no riding)	324
Painting the house	342
Ping pong	270
Playing cards	117
Playing piano	189
Racquetball	441
Raking leaves	342
Rearranging furniture	450
Rock climbing (ascending)	747
Rock climbing (repelling)	549
Roller skating/blading	477
Rowing	720
Rugby	684
Shoveling snow	405
Sledding	477
Snow skiing (cross-country)	549
Snow skiing (downhill)	441
Soccer	468

Activity (60 minutes)	Calories (150# person)
Spinning	477
Stacking firewood	414
Stair climbing	612
Surfing	207
Swimming	288
Swing dancing	270
Tae Kwon Do	342
Tai Chi	270
Tennis (doubles)	342
Tennis (singles)	549
Touch football	549
Volleyball (beach)	576
Walking (brisk)	297
Walking (stroll)	207
Washing the car	306
Washing the dishes	153
Watching TV	72
Water aerobics	288
Water polo	720
Water skiing	432
Weight lifting	207
Whitewater rafting	360
Working out at gym	378
Yoga	270

Table 9. Caloric Expenditure for Various Activities

Make sure you wear the right shoes (if you choose to begin a walking program, I would recommend a good pair of running shoes), wear comfortable clothing and are appropriately hydrated (drinking an 8-oz glass of water right before exercise, an 8-oz glass of water every 15 minutes during exercise and another 8-oz glass of water right after fin-ishing exercise).

Stretch the involved muscle groups for several minutes following your walk or other form of physical activity. About 10 to 20% of the total duration of your exercise should be spent stretching. Do each stretching exercise three to five times. Slowly stretch into the desired position (as far as possible without pain), hold the stretch for 15 to 30 seconds, relax, then repeat, trying to stretch even farther. Stretching helps: 1) improve performance; 2) reduce risk of injury; 3) relieve muscle soreness; 4) enhance posture; 5) increase blood supply to the tissues; 6) improve coordination; 7) reduce stress; and 8) make exercise more enjoyable.

When doing muscle strengthening exercises, don't hold your breath. Breathe out as you contract your muscles (push or pull weight) and breathe in as you relax them. Use smooth and steady movements rather than jerking or thrusting ones. Don't ever lock the joints of your arms or legs into a strained position. Take three seconds to push or pull a weight into place. Hold that position for one second then take another three sec-onds to lower the weight. Don't let the weight drop—lowering it slowly is real important.

Depending on how physically fit you are, you might need to start out with only minimal resistance (as little as one or two pounds of weight) to allow your muscles to adapt. Starting out with excessive resistance can lead to injuries. Use minimal resistance the first week then gradually increase as tolerated.

The resistance should feel hard for you but not very, very hard. If you can't push or pull a weight eight times in a row, it's too heavy for you. If you can push or pull a weight more than 15 times in a row, it's too light for you. Remember you must continue to increase the resistance over time in order to continue benefiting from muscle strengthening exercises. If you don't keep challenging your muscles, they won't get any stronger. About 20 to 30% of the total duration of your exercise should be spent doing muscle strengthening.

Remember to stretch the involved muscle groups for several minutes before doing muscle strengthening exercises after at least five minutes of 'warm up' aerobic activity. Stretching 'cold' muscles can lead to injury.

I would recommend you consider purchasing Thera-Band latex (or latex-free) exercise bands and/or rubber exercise tubing for upper body as well as lower body strengthening that include handles, door anchors and attachment devices. They come in up to eight different color-coded levels of resistance and are great for use at home, the office or while traveling (I use them when I travel since they're so convenient and allow me to get in a great workout almost anywhere).

Realize the more active you are, the more calories you get to consume. And since exercise leads to the breakdown of glycogen (a storage product made from sugar) within skeletal muscle, the more you exercise, the more natural sugars you get to eat—a small amount (e.g. one apple, banana or pear) by itself right before exercise and a larger amount along with some protein within 30 minutes following exercise (equivalent to the total calories burned during exercise [60–75% from high-GI carbohydrates and 25–40% from protein]). So if you feel like having a bowl of healthy cereal tonight (such as All-Bran or Kashi) with some blueberries and skim milk, you must first <u>EARN IT</u> by taking a brisk walk, getting on the treadmill or exercise bike, jumping rope, etc…

Recognize that your cravings for 'junk' food are usually due to an elevated insulin level (pathologic), and exercise is a great way (physiologic) to lower that level. So your desire for 'junk' is not a natural response to your body actually 'needing' any more calories or sugar. Here's how you can prove this to yourself. The next time you crave some sweet, starchy and/or salty 'junk' food, go take a brisk walk or bike ride (for <u>AT LEAST</u> 15 minutes) and make sure you build up a sweat. When you return home, the <u>LAST</u> thing on your mind will be consuming any junk. Think about it, if your body really needed those extra calories, and you just burnt off a bunch of them with exercise, you should want the junk more and not less. But, since your cravings were not normal and instead related to abnormal elevations of blood insulin, and exercise just lowered these— voilà, you don't want the junk after exercise because you didn't really need it in the first place. In fact, it wasn't even you who craved it; it was your pancreas (through its inappropriate release of insulin).

Chapter Six

HAPI Diet Principle #4: 'Exercise Smarter'

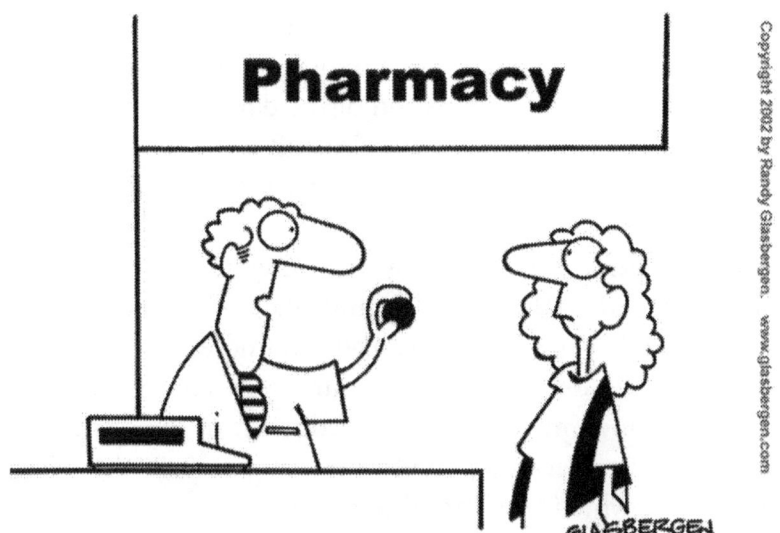

"It's the most effective diet pill we sell.
Chase it around a handball court for an hour a day."

Eat Earlier, Exercise Later,
Get Enough Sleep & 'Chill Out'

Probably the most beneficial thing you can do in losing weight (and the one with which most people have significant problem) is optimizing your body's BMR. The body goes through what is termed a 'circadian rhythm' when it comes to its daily metabolism—starting somewhat slow in the early morning when we are just awakening, becoming faster and faster as the day progresses, peaking in the early to mid-afternoon then slowing down once again as the evening commences to reach its nadir while we are fast asleep. Therefore, the body is at its most 'energy efficient' late in the evening, is somewhat energy efficient early in the morning but is very 'energy inefficient' in early to mid-afternoon. One useful trick in modifying your own BMR to enhance weight loss is to exercise when your body's metabolism would otherwise be diminished (in the evening and/or early morning) in order to 'speed things up' during that 'slow' period of the day and to eat the majority of your calories when your body's metabolism is enhanced (in early to mid-afternoon) in order to burn off most of those excess calories during that 'fast' period of the day. You thus receive maximal metabolic benefit from your exercise and minimal metabolic detriment from your caloric consumption. Try it…it really works.

One major benefit of working out first thing in the morning is to 'get it out of the way.' Most people will admit that if they put off exercising until later in the day, they're just as likely to find excuses why to 'put it off until tomorrow.' Also, if you begin your day in a healthy manner with exercise, you're much more likely to continue it in the same fashion—much less likely to overindulge with junk and reverse the wholesome momentum with which you started the day.

Eating frequent, relatively small meals has a major advantage in that it promotes optimal metabolism. Digesting food obviously burns off calories so the more frequent meals you consume the higher your BMR will be. Remember that one of the <u>WORST</u> things to do is skip breakfast and lunch and then have a large, late dinner.

Please also recognize the importance of a 'good night's rest.' The body (like all natural entities) functions on the principles of balance and homeostasis. Realize that your body demands a certain amount of sleep from you on a daily basis (obviously everyone is different—some people may need only five hours of sleep per day while others may require ten hours of sleep). If your body doesn't receive the amount of sleep it requires, important things related to your BMR will change during the waking hours so that your body eventually gets what it demands. You will tend to feel sleepier during the day (thus having a lower BMR and reducing your daily caloric expenditure) and you will tend to feel hungrier (thus probably increasing your daily caloric intake) with cravings mainly for refined, high-GI carbohydrates (which will increase your insulin level and further diminish your BMR).

Another thing to focus on is reducing your personal stress level. Remember that stress is how you respond to your situation (whether personal, financial, occupational or other) rather than the situation itself. The stress response alters many things in the human physiology, including elevating bloodstream cortisol levels which slow down BMR and promote the development of fat within the abdominal cavity, thus turning on the 'malignant' CE circuit. What can be done?

1) Live a lifestyle you can afford and don't value any goods or services more than your own sanity. Appreciate them for what they are and nothing more. Money should provide security and freedom—not enslave you. If you focus yourself on getting and/or accumulating better and better 'things,' you will never be happy since there always is a bigger house, faster car, larger bank account, etc...

2) Focus yourself on self-improvement, learning every day, following what you believe to be the truth and especially on improving those individuals around you. There are two main ways of feeling better about yourself: putting others down to feel superior for a moment (and your mother would be ashamed); or elevating others to feel better about yourself forever (and your mother would be proud).

3) Understand the power of breathing. How long could you live without food? A: weeks. How long could you live without water? A: days. How long could you live without air? A: minutes. We rarely concern ourselves with breathing since it is automatic. Whenever you feel stress, close your eyes, inhale deeply and slowly through your nostrils, fill your chest cavity with air, hold it for a second or two and then exhale slowly through your mouth. Repeat once or twice more. Now, don't you feel better?

4) Recognize the power of the human touch. We need to touch others and be touched ourselves in return. Why do you think monkeys and other primates are always grooming each other? It promotes social bonds and reduces stress. Once or twice a day, get a massage (focusing on the palms, soles, scalp, neck and low back) from your significant other and return the favor (and not just as a prelude to intercourse). If you don't have a significant other, go to a good massage therapist once or twice a week. If you can't afford such luxuries, give yourself a massage (focusing on the palms, soles and scalp) once or twice a day. If you find a spot that hurts, keep rubbing until it feels better.

5) Don't worry about things you can't control. Worry never helps anything, only makes you feel miserable and actually increases the odds things will not turn out in your favor. Instead trust your gut and your intuition. Remember that intuition isn't always right but when you don't listen to it, it's <u>ALWAYS</u> right.

6) Focus on the <u>NOW</u> and don't dwell in a past you can't change or plan neurotically and obsessively for a future that won't turn out the way you envision anyway. Don't be a robot just going through the motions within your own life. The only way to ensure both a favorable past and desirable future is to make the most of the now. Live every moment to its fullest, sucking the sweet juice from the fruit of life that could be plucked from your grasp at any moment.

7) Love and respect yourself. You can never truly love and/or respect others until you start with yourself. Don't be so hard on yourself, give yourself a break more often than not and realize you are only human (like everyone else) and thus fallible. We all have our warts, burps and farts. Learn and grow because of them not just despite them. In most cultures, the symbol of love is the heart—it should be no surprise that love (of oneself and of others) is thus the best answer to keep that heart as healthy as possible.

♟

Pressure Point Techniques to Suppress Appetite

Whenever I bring up the concept of considering Traditional Chinese Medicine (TCM) techniques, many patients seem reluctant and quite skeptical. I understand this quite well (as I used to feel the same) since TCM originates from a completely different culture, with a different belief and value system as well as a different way of looking at life, health, sickness and the human body. However, I will ask any skeptical individual three questions: 1) Do you think individuals of Chinese origin are genetically inferior in terms of their intelligence? (answer: NO!); 2) Do you think the Chinese culture is worthless, pathetic and has no value whatsoever? (answer: emphatic NO!!); and 3) Therefore, do you really think that over one billion intelligent people from an advanced culture have believed things about the human body for over 5000 years and it's all just 'smoke and mirrors'? (answer: emphatic <u>NO WAY</u>!!!).

Copyright 1996 by Randy Glasbergen.

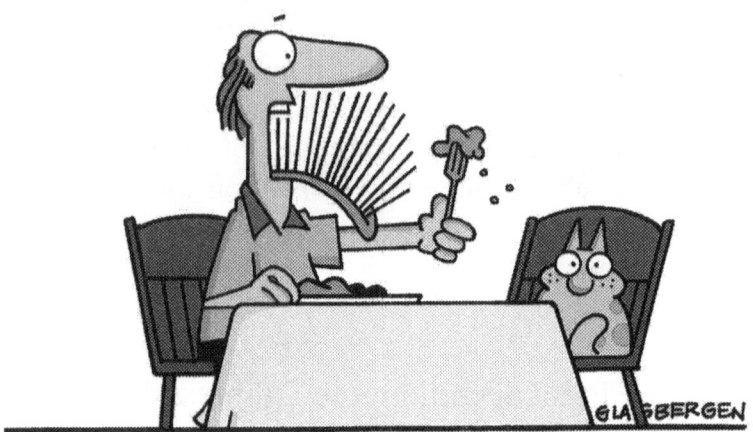

After years of unsuccessful weight loss programs, Burton lost 100 pounds on The Acupuncture Diet.

I have used the following two techniques (based on TCM acupuncture points) on myself many times and they do seem to work. Most patients who have tried them also agree that they were helpful in diminishing their cravings. 1) Place the tip of either your index or middle finger (whichever feels more natural) just beneath the tip of your nose right above the central groove of the upper lip. Press inward against the upper jaw and rotate in a circular motion for about ten seconds. Stop for a moment then repeat as needed (maybe two to four more times) to suppress the appetite. 2) Insert the tips of your index fingers gently into your ears (see Image 27 below), palms facing your cheeks. Place your thumbs on each antitragus (located just above the earlobes) and apply squeezing, rolling pressure to these flaps with both the thumbs (below) and index fingers (above) for about one minute. Then use your middle fingers to put pressure on the small bony indentations just anterior to each tragus with a circular motion for about one minute each.

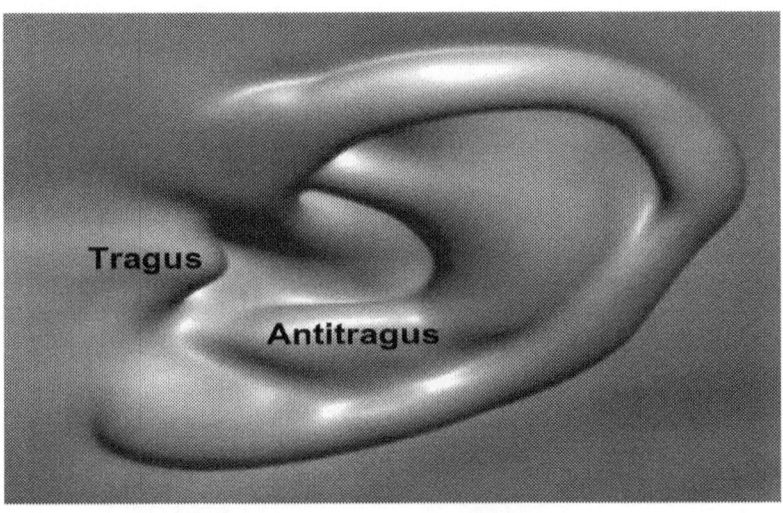

Image 27. Auricular Anatomy

Chapter Seven
HAPI Diet Principle #5:
'Have the Right Attitude'

Copyright 2004 by Randy Glasbergen.
www.glasbergen.com

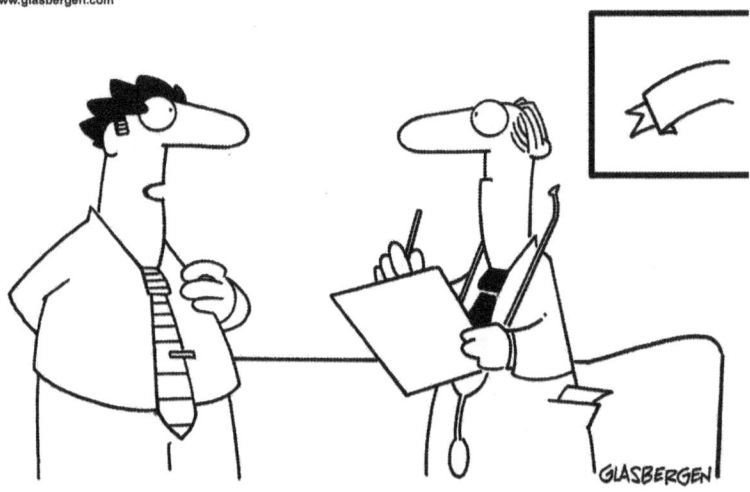

**"Diets don't work with my personality type.
I'm a winner, not a loser!"**

'I <u>Have to</u>, I <u>Want to</u> and I <u>WILL</u> Lose Weight'

In order to even consider losing weight, you must have the appropriate mind set: 'I have to, I want to and I will.' If you don't believe that you

HAVE TO lose weight, it won't happen. If you don't really WANT TO lose weight, it definitely won't happen. If you don't tell yourself that you WILL lose the weight, it also won't happen. If you instead simply set out to 'try' to lose weight, you're bound to fail. Trying implies the possibility and even the inevitability of failure. You either 'do it' or you try to do it. There is no middle ground. You must realize that if you set your mind to it and do what you need to do, there is no way you will fail in your goal of losing weight. Like many other important and valuable things in life, you need to decide whether to be a WINNER, a WIENER or a WHINER. In life, you either 'make things happen' for you or you 'allow things to happen' to you. You must attack weight loss the same way you have any other important and valuable thing in your life. Why can't it be easy? It can't be easy because NOTHING worth anything comes easy. All things of true value necessitate hard work. You can't count on luck—in fact you make your own luck if you really think about it. Why was Michael Jordan so 'lucky' on the basketball court? It's because he worked so hard at it off the basketball court, of course. The return on this investment is well worth it—I promise you. But it's your choice and it's your life.

♟

Patience and Perseverance are Virtues

There's a good reason it is said that 'patience is a virtue'…because it is. You must recognize that you didn't gain weight 'overnight' so there's no reason to believe that you must lose it overnight. As long as you recognize your ultimate goal of losing weight, never give up and make steady progress toward it (no matter how slow) you will definitely achieve that goal. You want your life to be more like a bottle of great Vintage Port (keeps improving as the years progress) rather than a bottle of Beaujolais (tastes OK today then rapidly turns into vinegar). Would you rather have the greatest day in your life today then everything goes downhill, or an average day today but things keep getting better and better over time?

A good idea is to set up multiple 'mini-goals' along your way to give yourself positive reinforcement—the first five pounds then the first 10 pounds then the first 15 pounds, etc...Imagine someone trying to learn how to pole vault for the first time: their initial goal is obviously not going to be 20 feet but rather one foot—followed by two feet then three feet, etc...Remember that the main difference between a winner and a wiener is that if the winner makes a mistake in progressing toward their goal, they recognize it as a such (just a minor mistake), correct it, learn from it and continue to move forward with even that much more determination and perseverance. On the other hand, if the wiener makes a mistake in progressing toward their goal, they view it as proof of their ultimate failure and just give up. Life is like an amusement park ride—you can make yours a Ferris wheel or a roller coaster. Ferris wheels (wieners) go up and down (like life does) but go nowhere. Roller coasters (winners) also go up and down but are constantly moving forward—with the momentum of falling giving them the ability to achieve even greater heights. Remember what Nietzsche said, "that what does not kill you makes you stronger." That is, <u>IF</u> you let it.

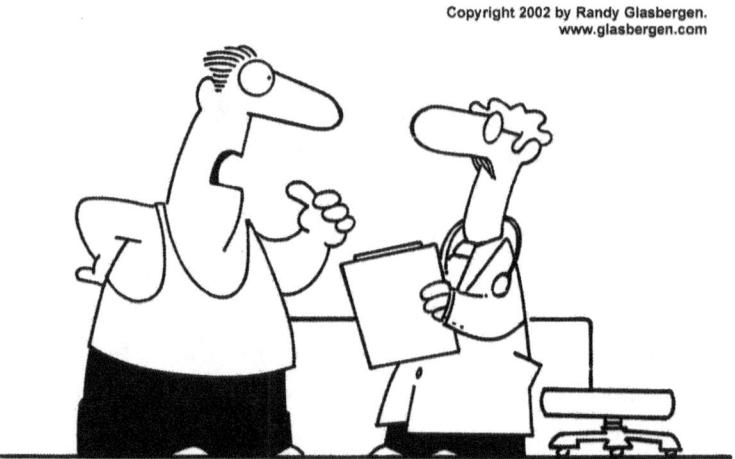

Copyright 2002 by Randy Glasbergen.
www.glasbergen.com

"I've always been a high achiever, always striving for bigger, faster, greater...and now suddenly I'm expected to settle for *lower* blood pressure and *less* cholesterol?!"

♟

Positive Thoughts Lead to Positive Outcome

Realize that negative thoughts breed negative outcomes whereas positive thoughts yield positive outcomes. If you notice that little voice inside your mind berating you with negative messages or making up excuses for your 'bad' behavior ("you're fat," "you're never going to lose weight," "you'll just gain it all back," "but I love chocolate," "I'm too tired to take a walk"), force yourself to turn the situation on its head with a positive spin and flood your mind with positive reinforcement ("I may be heavy now but just you wait," "I'm definitely going to lose this weight," "I'm going to keep the weight off this time," "chocolate's not that big a deal," "I'll feel great about myself after the walk"). Tell yourself these positive messages over and over again and eventually you <u>WILL</u> believe them. Brainwash yourself.

Another great technique is to visualize yourself in the future when you are lean and health-conscious. Whenever you plan to eat or exercise, really focus on this image and ask yourself: "What would the future lean, health-conscious me do?" and do that. Role-play that future slender you and you'll 'morph' yourself into that person sooner than you think. Since all people (kids as well as adults) love playing games, whenever you sit down to eat or get ready to begin your exercise routine, challenge yourself, "How can I do this in the best way to promote metabolism and lose weight?" Make eating and exercise fun. If you truly enjoy something, you'll excel in it; if you never really enjoy something, you'll never do it well.

♟

Losing Weight is a Job That <u>Must</u> Be Done Every Single Day

Think of your weight loss program as a job that <u>MUST</u> be done every single day for the rest of your life. Your intent is not just to lose weight in the short-term but rather to keep the weight off for the long run and thus promote a happy and healthy life. Before you can get a 'vacation' from your job (for Thanksgiving, Christmas, Easter, another major holiday, a wedding, a dinner party, etc…), you must prove yourself at your job as a good and productive employee. Remember you are proving yourself to yourself—at this job you are both employee as well as employer. Your job consists only of three distinct tasks: 1) decreasing caloric intake; 2) increasing caloric expenditure; and 3) optimizing BMR. That's it. The central trick to weight loss is changing certain of your 'bad' and self-destructive habits into 'good' and self-promoting ones. And realize that, all habits are 'hard to break,' including the good ones. These habits (good or bad) are just learned associations (like Dr. Pavlov's dog and the bell) that can be 'unlearned' if we put in the effort. If you crave a bowl of ice cream before going to bed, you must realize that eating that bowl tonight fuels the desire for it tomorrow night. Force yourself to avoid it for a few nights, and you won't even want it anymore (as long as you keep avoiding it).

The three tasks mentioned above will definitely lead to success—the only questions are how much focus and effort you must apply to each and how much time it will take. This is a battle between your positive self and your negative self. In such a battle, your positive self <u>CAN NOT LOSE</u> as long as it is appropriately armed ('eat less and eat smarter'), appropriately trained ('exercise more and exercise smarter') and appropriately motivated ('have the right attitude'—a <u>POSITIVE</u> one). It might take some time, but so what? Once you have altered your lifestyle sufficiently in order to lead to steady, persistent weight loss and once you feel secure of the inevitable success of your personalized weight loss program, then and only then can you take a 'vacation' from your job. A word of advice—for as much 'fun' as you have on your 'vacation,' that's how much work that will have 'piled up' upon your desk when you return to work.

Copyright 2003 by Randy Glasbergen.
www.glasbergen.com

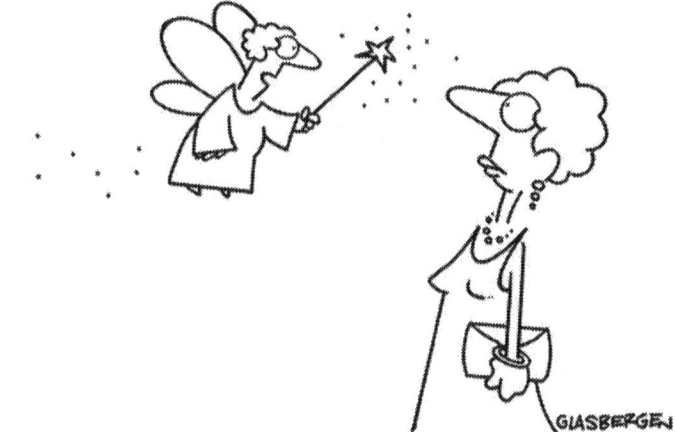

**"Have fun at the party, but remember —
at midnight you turn back into a dieter!"**

Chapter Eight
Recipes for the HAPI Heart

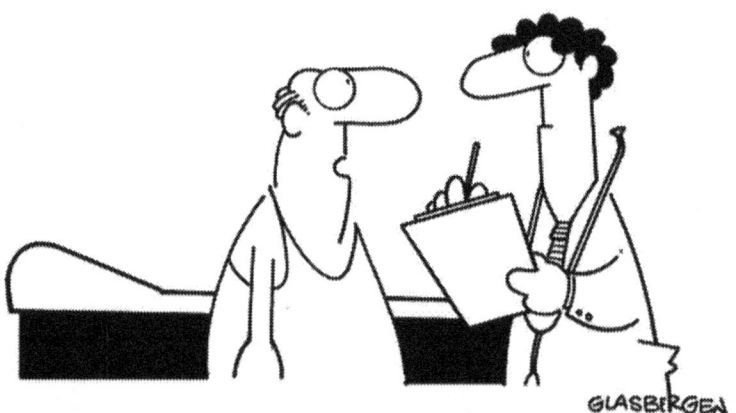

Copyright 2005 by Randy Glasbergen.
www.glasbergen.com

GLASBERGEN

"I tried the South Beach Diet, but I didn't read the book.
For two weeks I ate nothing but sand."

In this chapter, I've included some of my favorite recipes (with wine suggestions), modified to fit the principles of the HAPI Heart Diet. I hope you enjoy preparing, serving and eating them. Bon Appétit.

Part I. Getting Started

♟

HAPI Spice Mixture

Makes ½ cup

1½ T. garlic powder
1½ T. onion powder
1 T. ground red pepper
1 T. ground cinnamon
1 T. ground ginger
1 T. ground sweet paprika
1 T. ground turmeric

Combine the above ingredients together. May store in a closed container in a cool, dry place for 2 weeks before use.

♟

Vegetable Stock

Makes 4 cups

6 cups fresh cold water
2 medium yellow onions, quartered
2 leeks, white and tender green parts only, cleaned thoroughly and halved lengthwise
2 large carrots, peeled and halved
2 large celery stalks
1 small turnip, peeled and halved
8 garlic cloves, peeled and halved
8 oz. cremini mushrooms, halved
1 bay leaf
1 handful fresh parsley, including stems
1 handful fresh thyme, including stems

¼ cup celery leaves, torn
1 T. whole black peppercorns
1 T. whole coriander seeds

Combine all the above in a large stockpot over high heat, bring just to the start of a boil then lower the heat to a simmer for about 60 minutes. Strain into a clean pot then allow to cool, Either refrigerate until ready to use or place in ice cube trays, freeze then store in plastic freezer bags for later use (8 cubes equals 1 cup of stock).

♟

Roasted Vegetable Stock

Use same ingredients as above recipe. Preheat oven to 400° F. Lightly grease a roasting pan with some macadamia nut oil (www.oilsofaloha.com). Toss above ingredients up to and including the mushrooms in prepared pan and roast until well browned, about 1 hour. Remove the vegetables to a large stockpot, then deglaze the roasting pan with 1 cup of white wine or dry vermouth, scraping up any browned bits and then adding to the stockpot along with the bay leaf, parsley, thyme, celery leaves, peppercorns and coriander seeds. Add water, bring just to a boil then simmer for 60 minutes, strain and store for future use as per previous recipe.

♟

Basic Brown Sauce

Makes 4 cups

In a large, heavy saucepan, heat 3 T. extra-virgin olive oil and 3 T. macadamia nut oil over medium heat. Add ½ cup finely chopped yellow onion, ¼ cup finely chopped carrot and ¼ cup finely chopped celery and cook until caramelized. Add 6 T. whole wheat flour and cook, constantly stirring to make a brown roux, about 10 minutes. Gradually stir in 8 cups roasted vegetable stock, 2 cups chopped fresh tomatoes, 1 bay leaf, 1 handful fresh parsley (including stems), 1 handful fresh thyme (including stems), ¼ cup torn celery leaves, 4 whole cloves and 4 allspice berries. Bring just to the start of a boil then lower the heat to a bare simmer for about 2 hours, stirring occasionally. The final sauce should be the consistency of a heavy cream. Strain and store for future use as per previous recipes.

☖

Sauce Demi-Glace

Makes 4 cups

Combine 4 cups Basic Brown Sauce, 4 cups Roasted Vegetable Stock and 1 cup chopped cremini mushrooms in a large stockpot over medium heat. Bring just to the start of a boil then lower the heat to a bare simmer until cooked down by half, about 2 hours. Strain into a clean saucepan, stir in ½ cup port, Madeira or dry sherry then store for future use as per previous recipes.

♟

Part II. Soup
☖
Wild Mushroom Soup

Serves: 4

1 medium yellow onion, peeled and sliced
3 garlic cloves, peeled and halved
½ cup extra-virgin olive oil (or ¼ cup olive oil plus ¼ cup macadamia nut oil)
2 T. Madras curry powder
½ T. ground thyme
16 oz white button mushrooms, cleaned and halved
4 cups Roasted Vegetable Stock (see above recipe)

8 oz assorted wild mushrooms (chanterelle, morel, oyster, shitake), thickly sliced
2 garlic cloves, peeled and minced
2 T. fresh thyme leaves
Fresh ground black pepper, to taste

In a large heavy saucepan, heat ¼ cup of the olive oil over medium heat; add the onions, halved garlic, curry powder and ground thyme. Cook until the onion is translucent, about 10 minutes. Add the white mushrooms and cook until all the vegetables are tender, about 20 minutes more. Add the stock, increasing the heat just to the start of a boil then lower to a simmer over medium-low heat for about 30 minutes. Let cool slightly then purée in batches in a food processor or blender. Return to the stockpot and keep warm.

Meanwhile, heat the remaining olive oil in a medium sauté pan over medium-high heat. Add the wild mushrooms, minced garlic and thyme leaves, season with some black pepper and cook until the mushrooms are starting to brown, about 7 minutes.

Ladle some soup into each soup bowl. Spoon some wild mushrooms on top in the center, season with some black pepper and serve immediately. Great with Californian or Australian Chardonnay or white Burgundy.

PER SERVING
Calories: 304
Protein (grams): 2
Fat: 28
Carbohydrates: 11
Fiber: 3

♟

Butternut Squash and Leek Soup

Serves: 4

2 T. extra-virgin olive oil (or 1 T. olive oil plus 1 T. macadamia nut oil)
4 leeks, white and tender green parts only, cleaned thoroughly and coarsely chopped
1 celery stalk, chopped
1 medium carrot, peeled and chopped
2 garlic cloves, peeled and halved
4 cups Roasted Vegetable Stock (see above recipe)
1 medium tomato, chopped
1 large butternut squash, peeled and cut into large dice
1 bay leaf
¼ cup fresh flat-leaf parsley leaves
½ cup nonfat plain yogurt
Fresh ground black pepper, to taste

Heat the olive oil in a large, heavy saucepan. Add the leeks, celery, carrot and garlic and cook over moderate heat for about 7 minutes, until the vegetables have softened. Add the stock, tomato, squash and bay leaf, increase the heat just to the start of a boil then reduce to a simmer over moderate-low heat until the vegetables are quite tender, about 25 minutes. Discard the bay leaf and stir in the parsley.

Let cool slightly then purée in batches in a food processor or blender. Return to the saucepan, warm to a simmer then stir in the yogurt. Ladle some soup into each soup bowl. Season with the black pepper and serve immediately. Great with Californian Chenin Blanc or Vouvray.

PER SERVING
Calories: 177
Protein (grams): 4

Fat: 9
Carbohydrates: 20
Fiber: 4

☖

Asparagus-Avocado Vichyssoise

Serves: 4

2 T. extra-virgin olive oil (or 1 T. olive oil plus 1 T. macadamia nut oil)
2 leeks, white and tender green parts only, cleaned thoroughly and sliced
4 cups Vegetable Stock (see above recipe)
2 lbs. asparagus, tips cut to 1 inch, tender parts of stalk chopped (rough parts of stem discarded)
3 cups baby spinach leaves
1 fresh, ripe avocado, halved, cored and coarsely chopped
¼ cup nonfat plain yogurt
Fresh ground black pepper, to taste

Heat the olive oil in a medium saucepan. Add the leeks and cook over moderate-low heat until softened, about 6 minutes. Add the stock and chopped asparagus stems, increase the heat just to the start of a boil then reduce to a simmer over medium-low heat and cook for about 6 minutes, until the stems become tender. Add the spinach and avocado and cook for 3 minutes.

Let cool slightly then purée in batches in a food processor or blender. Season with some black pepper, then refrigerate until chilled, about 2 hours.

Bring water to a boil in a medium saucepan then add the asparagus tips and cook until crisp-tender, about 3 minutes. Remove with slotted spoon and place in bowl of ice water for about 1 minute. Drain then pat dry.

Ladle some soup into each soup bowl, stir 1 T. yogurt into each then spoon some of the asparagus tips on top. Season with some black pepper and serve. Great with Californian, Australian, New Zealand or Chilean Sauvignon Blanc, Sancerre or dry white Bordeaux.

PER SERVING
Calories: 355
Protein (grams): 10
Fat: 23
Carbohydrates: 27
Fiber: 9

♟

Spicy Vegetarian Chili

Serves: 4

2 T. extra-virgin olive oil (or 1 T. olive oil plus 1 T. macadamia nut oil)
½ cup chopped peeled carrots
½ cup chopped red bell peppers
½ cup chopped green bell peppers
½ cup chopped onions
2 cloves garlic, peeled and minced
1 fresh Serrano pepper, cored, seeded and finely chopped
1 T. ground chili powder
½ T. ground cayenne pepper
½ T. ground cumin
14 oz. can plum tomatoes, with juice, coarsely chopped
8 oz. can red kidney beans, soaked and rinsed multiple times to remove salt
8 oz. can cannellini beans, soaked and rinsed multiple times to remove salt
8. oz can black beans, soaked and rinsed multiple times to remove salt
½ cup bold red wine (Californian Zinfandel or Australian Shiraz)

¼ cup nonfat yogurt
¼ cup fresh cilantro leaves and tender stems, coarsely chopped
Fresh ground black pepper, to taste

Heat the olive oil in a large saucepan. Add the carrots, bell peppers, onions and garlic and cook over medium heart until the onions turn golden, about 12 minutes. Add the Serrano pepper, chili powder, cayenne pepper and cumin and cook for 2 minutes. Add the plum tomatoes, all the beans and the red wine, bring just to the start of a boil then reduce to medium-low heat and simmer for about 45 minutes.

Ladle some chili into each soup bowl, stir 1 T. yogurt into each and sprinkle 1 T. cilantro leaves on top. Season with the black pepper and serve immediately. Great with Californian Zinfandel, Australian Shiraz, Côte du Rhône, Chianti Classico or Rioja.

PER SERVING
Calories: 345
Protein (grams): 15
Fat: 15
Carbohydrates: 51
Fiber: 15

♟

Niki's Gazpacho

Serves: 4

2 lbs. ripe tomatoes, cored and coarsely chopped
1 medium cucumber, peeled and coarsely chopped
1 medium green bell pepper, cored, peeled, seeded and coarsely chopped
2 cloves garlic, peeled and coarsely chopped
¼ cup red wine vinegar

¼ cup extra-virgin olive oil (preferably Spanish)
3 T. packed fresh parsley (or cilantro) leaves and tender stems
Fresh black pepper, to taste

Place the tomatoes in a food processor or blender and purée. With the machine running, add the cucumber, bell pepper, garlic, vinegar, olive oil and parsley leaves in succession until well blended. Let cool in the refrigerator for at least 2 hours. Ladle some gazpacho into each chilled soup bowl, season with the black pepper and serve.

PER SERVING
Calories: 258
Protein (grams): 3
Fat: 14
Carbohydrates: 20
Fiber: 3

Part III. Salad

Copyright 2002 by Randy Glasbergen.
www.glasbergen.com

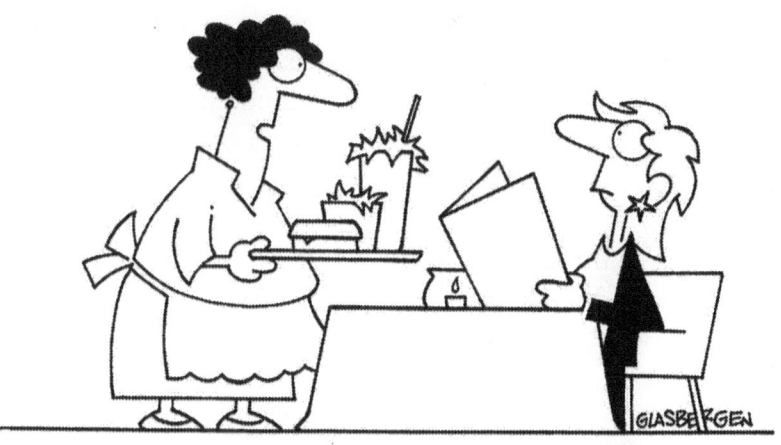

**"Our diet special is a fresh garden salad
served in burger, shake and fry containers."**

Ā

Festive Greek Salad

Serves: 4

4 cups mixed baby salad greens
2 cups baby spinach leaves
1 yellow bell pepper, cored, halved and cut into ¼ inch strips
1 red bell pepper, cored, halved and cut into ¼ inch strips
1 European-style cucumber, peeled and diced
1 medium red onion, peeled and diced
4 large ripe tomatoes, cored and diced
½ cup extra-virgin olive oil (preferably Greek)
¼ cup fresh lemon juice
1 T. pomegranate molasses
1 t. ground oregano (or more to taste)
1. t. ground white pepper (or more to taste)
8 Greek cracked green olives, soaked and rinsed multiple times to remove salt
12 Kalamata olives, soaked and rinsed multiple times to remove salt
¼ lb. crumbled non-fat Feta cheese, soaked in water to remove salt
Fresh ground black pepper, to taste

In a large bowl, combine the salad greens and baby spinach with the bell peppers, cucumber, red onion and tomatoes. In a small bowl, whisk the olive oil with the lemon juice and pomegranate molasses; season with the ground oregano and ground white pepper. Add the dressing to the salad and toss.

Place a portion of the salad onto the center of each plate. Top each with 2 cracked green and 3 Kalamata olives. Sprinkle some feta on top, season with the black pepper and serve.

PER SERVING
Calories: 358

Protein (grams): 8
Fat: 22
Carbohydrates: 32
Fiber: 8

♟

Fresh Herb Salad with Avocado, Cranberries & Truffle Vinaigrette

Serves: 4

1 cup fresh herb leaves (any combination of basil, chervil, cilantro, marjoram, mint, parsley, sage and tarragon)
4 cups mixed baby salad greens
1 ripe avocado, halved, cored and sliced
¼ cup extra-virgin olive oil (or 2 T. olive oil plus 2 T. avocado oil)
¼ cup white truffle oil
¼ cup sherry vinegar
2 t. Dijon mustard
1 garlic clove, peeled and minced
1 small shallot, peeled and minced
2 T. dried cranberries (unsweetened)
Fresh ground black pepper, to taste

In a large bowl, combine the herb leaves with the salad greens. In a small bowl, combine the vinegar with the mustard, garlic and shallot and let stand for 5 minutes. Whisk in the oils, then add the dressing to the salad and toss well.

Place a portion of the salad onto the center of each plate. Top with some Avocado slices and sprinkle with dried cranberries. Season with the black pepper and serve.

PER SERVING
Calories: 209

Protein (grams): 4
Fat: 17
Carbohydrates: 13
Fiber: 4

⚑

Tomato-Basil Salad with Fried Shallots

Serves: 4

3 large shallots, peeled, halved and separated into rings
1 small shallot, peeled and minced
½ cup fresh basil leaves, thinly sliced plus 1 T. minced
1½ T. red wine vinegar
3 T. extra-virgin olive oil
1 cup macadamia nut oil
3 lbs. assorted fresh and ripe tomatoes, cored and sliced (or halved if cherry)
Fresh ground black pepper, to taste

In a small bowl, combine the minced shallot with the minced basil and vinegar and let stand for 5 minutes. Whisk in the olive oil then season with some black pepper.

Meanwhile, in a medium saucepan, heat the macadamia nut oil until shimmering. Add half the sliced shallots and cook over moderate-high heat, stirring occasionally until browned, about 5 minutes. Transfer to some paper towels to drain any excess oil. Repeat with the remaining shallots.

Layer some tomato slices neatly across the center of each plate. Place some fried shallots over top. Sprinkle with sliced basil, drizzle with the vinaigrette, season with some black pepper and serve.

PER SERVING
Calories: 183

Protein (grams): 4
Fat: 7
Carbohydrates: 26
Fiber: 5

Part IV. Pasta

Spaghetti with Feta, Olives & Green Beans

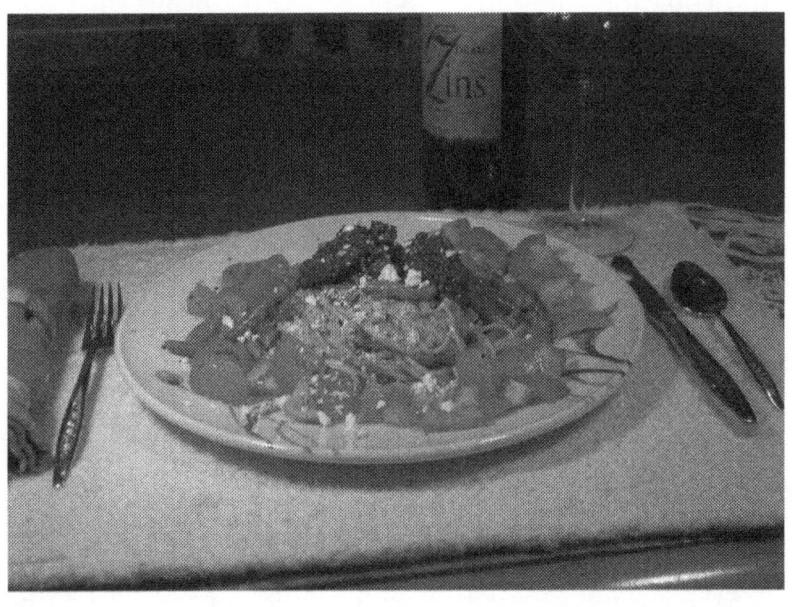

Serves: 4

1 lb. mixed fresh green and yellow beans
½ cup extra-virgin olive oil (or ¼ cup olive oil plus ¼ cup macadamia nut oil)
1 medium yellow onion, peeled and diced
6 large garlic cloves, peeled, 3 minced and 3 coarsely chopped
2/3 lb. 100% whole wheat spaghetti, dried

30 Kalamata olives, soaked and rinsed multiple times to remove salt, pitted and coarsely chopped
3 large tomatoes, cored and diced
3 T. fresh lemon juice
½ cup crumbled non-fat Feta cheese, soaked in water to remove salt
Fresh ground black pepper, to taste

Trim ends of green/yellow beans and slice at an angle into ½ inch pieces. In a small sauté pan, heat half of the olive oil over medium-low heat; add the onion and cook slowly into translucent. Add the minced garlic cloves and cook for one minute longer. Add the beans then cover the pan. Cook slowly for about 20 minutes, until the beans are beginning to soften. Season with some black pepper and keep warm.

Meanwhile, bring a large pot of water to a rolling boil. Add the spaghetti and cook for about 9–10 minutes until al dente. Drain well.

In one small bowl, combine the chopped olives with the chopped garlic. In another small bowl, toss the diced tomatoes with the lemon juice. Set both aside.

In a large sauté pan, heat the remaining olive oil over medium heat. Add the cooked pasta and toss.

Transfer a portion of pasta onto the center of each plate. Top with a mound of the green bean mixture with a dollop of the olive-garlic mixture on top. Surround the pasta with the tomato-lemon mixture. Sprinkle some feta on top, season with some black pepper and serve immediately. Great with Californian Zinfandel, Australian Shiraz, Côte du Rhône, Chianti Classico or Rioja.

PER SERVING
Calories: 512
Protein (grams): 11

Fat: 32
Carbohydrates: 45
Fiber: 7

♙

Linguini with Macadamia-Herb Pesto and Wilted Spinach

Serves: 4

1 cup packed fresh flat-leaf parsley leaves
1 cup packed fresh basil leaves
1 T. fresh mint leaves
1 T. fresh tarragon leaves
¼ cup raw macadamia nuts
2 T. sherry vinegar
¼ cup plus 2 T. extra-virgin olive oil
¼ cup macadamia nut oil
2/3 lb. 100% whole-wheat linguini, dried
2 cups fresh baby spinach leaves
Fresh ground black pepper, to taste

In a food processor, combine the parsley, basil, mint, tarragon, macadamia nuts, vinegar, macadamia nut oil and ¼ cup of the olive oil. Blend until a coarse purée forms then scrape into a small bowl and season with some black pepper.

Meanwhile, bring a large pot of water to a rolling boil. Add the linguini and cook for about 9–10 minutes until al dente. Reserve ¼ cup of the pasta cooking water then drain the linguini and place in large saucepan on low heat to keep warm.

Return the pasta pot to moderate-high heat. Add the remaining 2 T. olive oil and the spinach, stirring, until just wilted, about 30 seconds. Add the spinach to the pasta along with 3 T. of reserved pasta cooking water and the pesto. Toss with tongs to evenly distribute the spinach and pesto. Add the remaining 1 T. of reserved cooking water if the pasta seems dry.

Transfer a portion of pasta onto the center of each plate, season with some black pepper and serve immediately. Great with Californian, Australian, New Zealand or Chilean Sauvignon Blanc, Sancerre or dry white Bordeaux.

PER SERVING
Calories: 534
Protein (grams): 12
Fat: 34
Carbohydrates: 45
Fiber: 6

♟

Angel-Hair Pasta with Spicy Vegetable Ragout

Serves: 4

½ lb. fresh peas, shelled
2 large ripe tomatoes, cored
2 T. extra-virgin olive oil (or 1 T. olive oil plus 1 T. macadamia nut oil)
2 ears of corn, shucked, kernels cut off the cob
4 large scallions, white and tender green parts thinly sliced, dark green tops finely chopped
1 red bell pepper, cored, chopped into small dice
1 small zucchini, ends removed, chopped into small dice
3 large garlic cloves, peeled and minced
1 cup Roasted Vegetable Stock (see above recipe)
4 asparagus spears, peeled and cut into small dice (rough parts of stem discarded)
½ T. ground cayenne pepper
¼ cup packed fresh basil leaves, coarsely chopped

2/3 lb. 100% whole-wheat angel hair pasta, dried
Fresh ground black pepper, to taste

Bring a medium saucepan of water to a boil. Add the peas and cook until just tender, about 5 minutes. Remove with slotted spoon, place in bowl of ice water for about 1 minute then drain.

Return the water in the saucepan to a boil and add the tomatoes. Cook for 10 seconds then transfer to a bowl of ice water. Peel the tomatoes and cut in half. Working over a strainer set over a small bowl; scrape the seeds out with a spoon. Press on the seeds to extract their juice then discard them. Finely chop 1 of the tomatoes and add it to the tomato juice in the small bowl. Cut the other tomato into medium dice and set aside.

Heat half the olive oil in a large skillet. Add the corn, scallions, bell pepper, zucchini, garlic and peas and cook over moderate heat until softened, about 5 minutes. Add the stock and asparagus and cook until the liquid has been reduced by half, about 5 minutes. Stir in the contents of the small bowl and the cayenne pepper. Cook over moderate heat until most of the liquid has evaporated, about 3 minutes. Remove from the heat and stir in the basil, scallion tops and diced tomato.

Meanwhile, bring a large pot of water to a rolling boil. Add the angel hair pasta and cook for about 5–6 minutes until al dente. Drain well.

Toss the pasta with the remaining olive oil then transfer a portion of it onto the center of each plate. Top with some ragout, season with the black pepper and serve immediately. Great with Californian or Oregonian Pinot Noir or red Burgundy.

PER SERVING
Calories: 405
Protein (grams): 14
Fat: 9

Carbohydrates: 57
Fiber: 8

†

Part V. Fish
(Serve all Fish Entrées with Steamed/Sautéed Vegetables
or Small Green Salad and ½ Baked Sweet Potato or 1 Cup of
either Wild Rice or Whole Wheat Pasta)

Ꝕ

Pan-Roasted Salmon with Sun-Dried
Tomato-Kalamata Sauce

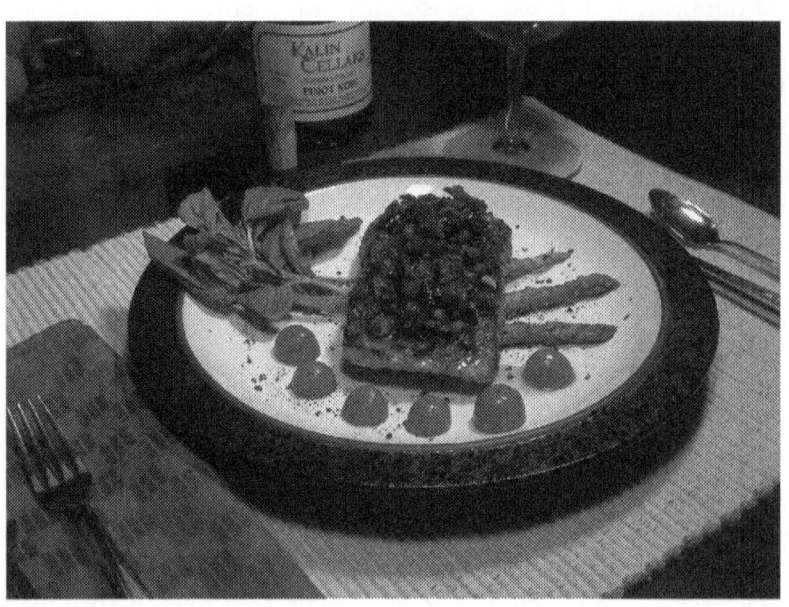

Serves: 4

2 T. capers, soaked and rinsed multiple times to remove salt
10 Kalamata olives, soaked and rinsed multiple times to remove salt, pitted and coarsely chopped

¼ cup sun-dried tomatoes (packed in extra-virgin olive oil), coarsely chopped
2 T. fresh basil leaves, finely chopped
2 garlic cloves, peeled and minced
2 T. extra-virgin olive oil
2 T. macadamia nut oil
1 T. ground onion powder
1 T. ground garlic powder
1 T. ground chili powder
4 6-oz salmon fillets (preferably wild coho), skin removed
1 T. high-quality liquid fish oil (optional—www.carlsonlabs.com)
Fresh ground black pepper, to taste

In a small bowl, combine the capers, kalamatas, sun-dried tomatoes, basil, garlic and olive oil. Heat a small skillet over medium heat. Add the contents of the small bowl, cook for about 4 minutes then return the contents to the small bowl and season with some black pepper.

Meanwhile, in a large skillet, heat the macadamia nut oil over moderate-high heat. Season both sides of the salmon fillets with the onion, garlic and chili powders then cook, about 3 minutes per side, until the fish is just cooked through.

Transfer one fillet onto the center of each plate. Top with some of the sautéed vegetables, drizzle with some fish oil, season with some black pepper and serve immediately. Great with Californian or Oregonian Pinot Noir or red Burgundy.

PER SERVING
Calories: 385
Protein (grams): 30
Fat: 25
Carbohydrates: 10
Fiber: 4

♟

Pan-Seared Salmon with Jalapeño-Avocado Vinaigrette

Serves: 4

2 T. apple cider vinegar
2 T. red onion, finely chopped
1 T. honey
1 T. fresh cilantro leaves, finely chopped
1 t. garlic, finely chopped
½ t. Dijon mustard
½ cup extra-virgin olive oil
1 T. macadamia nut oil
1 medium jalapeno
4 6-oz salmon fillets (preferably wild coho), skin removed
½ avocado, cored and diced
1 T. high-quality liquid fish oil (optional)
Fresh ground black pepper, to taste

In a small bowl, combine the vinegar and onion. Let stand for about 10 minutes, then whisk in the honey, cilantro, garlic, mustard and ¼ cup of olive oil.

Meanwhile, in a small skillet, heat the macadamia nut oil over high heat just until smoking. Add the jalapeño and cook, turning, until charred on all sides, about 2 minutes. Let cool then slip off the charred skin, discarding the stem and halving the jalapeño lengthwise. Spoon out the seeds, finely chop the jalapeño then stir into the vinaigrette, seasoning with some black pepper.

In a large skillet, heat the remaining olive oil over moderate-high heat. Season the salmon fillets with some black pepper and cook, about 3 minutes per side, until the fish is just cooked through.

Transfer one fillet onto the center of each plate. Whisk the vinaigrette one last time then toss in the avocado. Spoon this mixture over each fillet, drizzle with fish oil, season with some black pepper and serve immediately. Great with Californian or Australian Chardonnay or white Burgundy.

PER SERVING
Calories: 474
Protein (grams): 32
Fat: 30
Carbohydrates: 19
Fiber: 6

Å

Sautéed Swordfish with Shallot-Triple Herb Topping

Serves: 4

2 12-oz swordfish steaks, at least 1 inch thick, skin removed
½ cup whole wheat flour
2 T. HAPI spice mixture (see above recipe)
¼ cup extra-virgin olive oil (or 2 T. olive oil and 2 T. macadamia nut oil)
½ T. fresh basil leaves, coarsely chopped
½ T. fresh mint leaves, coarsely chopped
½ T. fresh tarragon leaves, coarsely chopped
¼ cup chopped shallot
½ cup fresh home-made breadcrumbs made from all-natural whole wheat bread
½ cup dry white Vermouth
1 T. high-quality liquid fish oil (optional)
Fresh ground black pepper, to taste

Preheat the oven to 375°F. On a plate, combine the whole wheat flour with the HAPI spice mixture. Dredge the swordfish steaks in the seasoned flour, shaking off any excess and season with some black pepper.

In a large skillet over moderate-high heat, brown the swordfish steaks lightly on both sides in the olive oil, about 2 to 3 minutes per side. Sprinkle the herbs and shallots over the fish then cover with a 1/8 inch layer of bread crumbs. Baste with the sautéing oil. Pour the Vermouth around the fish; it should come about halfway up the sides of the steaks.

Bake the swordfish for about 20 to 25 minutes in the oven, basting several times with the liquid in the skillet. Remove from the oven, cut each steak in half then transfer one piece to the center of each plate. Drizzle with the fish oil, season with some black pepper then serve immediately. Great with Californian, Australian, New Zealand or Chilean Sauvignon Blanc, Sancerre or dry white Bordeaux.

PER SERVING
Calories: 471
Protein (grams): 43
Fat: 23
Carbohydrates: 13
Fiber: 2

♟

Greek-Style Baked Swordfish 'Plaki'

Serves: 4

4 6-oz swordfish steaks, at least 1 inch thick, skin removed
¼ cup whole wheat flour
2 T. ground oregano
½ T. ground white pepper
2 medium ripe tomatoes, cored and cut crosswise into ¼-inch slices
1 medium red onion, peeled and cut crosswise into ¼-inch slices
2 lemons, rind and white pith removed, seeded and cut crosswise into ¼-inch slices

12 Kalamata olives, soaked and rinsed multiple times to remove salt, pitted and quartered lengthwise
½ cup crumbled non-fat Feta cheese, soaked in water to remove salt
¼ cup extra-virgin olive oil (preferably Greek)
Fresh black pepper to taste

Preheat the oven to 375°F. On a large plate, combine the flour, oregano and white pepper. Place the swordfish steaks into a large, ovenproof baking dish. Sprinkle some seasoned flour onto the top surface of the fish. Place a layer of tomatoes followed by onion and finally lemons on top of the swordfish steaks. Spread some olives followed by cheese on top, drizzle with olive oil, season with some black pepper and bake in the oven for about 30–35 minutes.

Remove from the oven, transfer one swordfish steak with its vegetable covering onto the center of each plate, season with some black pepper and serve immediately. Great with Californian, Australian, New Zealand or Chilean Sauvignon Blanc, Sancerre or dry white Bordeaux.

PER SERVING
Calories: 416
Protein (grams): 41
Fat: 16
Carbohydrates: 17
Fiber: 4

♟
Cod Marsala

Serves: 4

1 cup cremini mushrooms, quartered
¼ cup celery stalk, cut into medium dice
¼ cup carrot, peeled, cut into medium dice

½ cup onion, peeled, cut into medium dice
2 garlic cloves, peeled and minced
2 T. extra-virgin olive oil
2 T. macadamia nut oil
2 cups Roasted Vegetable Stock (see above recipe)
2 cups dry Marsala
4 6-oz fresh cod fillets
2 T. garlic powder
1 T. high-quality liquid fish oil (optional)
Fresh ground black pepper, to taste

In a large saucepan, heat the olive oil and add the mushrooms, celery, carrot, onion and garlic and cook over moderate-high heat until the vegetables are quite tender, about 8 minutes. Add the stock and Marsala, increase the heat to moderate-high and reduce to 2 cups of liquid, about another 5 minutes. Reduce the heat to low and keep warm.

Meanwhile, season both sides of the cod fillets with the garlic powder and some black pepper. Heat the macadamia nut oil in a large skillet, add the cod fillets and cook over moderate-high heat until just cooked through, about 2–3 minutes per side.

Transfer one cod fillet to the center of each plate. Pour some sauce and vegetables over top, drizzle with the fish oil, season with some black pepper and serve immediately. Great with Californian or Oregonian Pinot Noir or red Burgundy.

PER SERVING
Calories: 312
Protein (grams): 30
Fat: 16
Carbohydrates: 12
Fiber: 3

♟

Roasted Cod with Prosciutto and Sage

Serves: 4

2 medium carrots, peeled and cut into medium dice
2 T. extra-virgin olive oil (or 1 T. olive oil and 1 T. macadamia nut oil)
1 small yellow onion, peeled and finely diced
½ head of Savoy cabbage, finely shredded
2 T. fresh flat-leaf parsley, coarsely chopped
1 T. ground coriander
4 6-oz fresh cod fillets
12 fresh sage leaves, 8 whole and 4 minced
4 paper-thin slices prosciutto di Parma
2 T. whole wheat flour
1 cup dry white Vermouth
Juice and finely grated zest of 1 small lemon
1 cup Roasted Vegetable Stock (see above recipe)
2 T. extra-virgin olive oil
1 T. high-quality liquid fish oil (optional)
Fresh ground black pepper, to taste

Preheat oven to 400°F. In a small saucepan, boil the carrots in lightly salted water until just tender, about 2 minutes. Drain and rinse under cold water until cool. Set aside in small bowl.

In a large skillet, sauté the onion over moderate-high heat in 1 T. of the olive oil. Add the cabbage and toss to coat with oil. Reduce the heat to medium and cook, until softened, about 5 minutes. Stir in the parsley and coriander and season with some black pepper. Keep warm over very low heat. Pad the cod dry and place 2 whole sage leaves on top of each fillet. Wrap a slice of prosciutto around each fillet and secure with a wooden toothpick. Lightly dust the cod with flour and season with some black pepper.

Heat the remaining 1 T. olive oil in a large nonstick skillet. Cook the cod in batches over moderate-high heat until browned and crisp, about 2 to 3 minutes per side. Transfer the fillets to a small baking sheet using a spatula. Roast the fish in the oven until just cooked through, about 8 minutes.

Meanwhile, set the skillet in which the cod was browned over high heat. Add the Vermouth, lemon juice and lemon zest and bring to a boil, scraping up any browned bits from the bottom of the pan until just a few tablespoons of liquid remain, about 5 minutes. Add the stock, olive oil and reserved carrots and boil until reduced by half, about 5 minutes. Add the minced sage and season with some black pepper.

Mound some cabbage in the center of each plate. Place a piece of cod on top, discarding the toothpick. Spoon the sauce over the fish, drizzle with some fish oil, season with some black pepper and serve immediately. Great with Californian or Australian Chardonnay or white Burgundy.

PER SERVING
Calories: 354
Protein (grams): 35
Fat: 18
Carbohydrates: 13
Fiber: 2

♟

Nut-Crusted Sea Bass with Chanterelle Vinaigrette

Serves: 4

3 raw hazelnuts
3 raw almonds
3 raw macadamia nuts

2 T. coriander seeds
2 T. sesame seeds
1 T. whole black peppercorns
5 T. extra-virgin olive oil
1 cup Vegetable Stock (see above recipe)
1 oz package of dried chanterelle mushrooms
1 T. honey
1 T. fresh lemon juice
1 T. sherry vinegar
1 T. low-sodium soy sauce
½ cup whole what flour
4 egg whites
¼ cup macadamia nut oil
4 6-oz sea bass fillets, skinned
1 T. high-quality liquid fish oil (optional)
Fresh ground black pepper, to taste

In a small skillet, mix the hazelnuts, almonds, macadamia nuts, coriander seeds, sesame seeds and peppercorns. Toast over moderate-low heat until fragrant and slightly browned, about 4 minutes. Remove from the heat and let cool. Transfer the contents of the skillets to a spice grinder and grind to a coarse powder.

Place vegetable stock in medium pot, bring just a boil, remove from the heat, mix in the package of dried chanterelle mushrooms, cover and let sit for about 30 minutes. Strain into a clean pot and keep warm. Rinse the reconstituted mushrooms several times in fresh water to remove all grit then place between some paper towels and press firmly to remove all moisture.

Heat 1 T. of the olive oil in a large skillet, add the mushrooms and cook over moderate-high heat until nicely browned, about 8 minutes. Add the chanterelle liquid, honey, lemon juice, vinegar and soy sauce and bring to a boil over high heat. Reduce the heat to low and simmer for about 20 minutes, until the liquid has been reduced to about ¼ cup. Strain the mixture through a fine-mesh sieve into a small saucepan, pressing hard on the solids to remove as much liquid as possible. Whisk the remaining oil into the contents of the small saucepan and keep warm.

Spread the nut-spice powder on one plate and the flour on another. Coat the sea bass fillets with the nut-spice powder, dip into the egg whites then coat with the flour, shaking off any excess. In a large skillet, heat the macadamia nut oil and add 2 of the sea bass fillets, cooking over moderate heat until browned and just cooked through, about 4 minutes per side. Transfer the cooked fish to a warm platter and repeat with the remaining 2 fillets.

Transfer one sea bass fillet onto the center of each plate. Spoon some shitake vinaigrette on top, drizzle with the fish oil, season with the black pepper and serve immediately. Great with Californian or Australian Chardonnay or white Burgundy.

PER SERVING
Calories: 437
Protein (grams): 40
Fat: 21
Carbohydrates: 22
Fiber: 8

♟
Grilled Sea Bass with Rosemary and Thyme

Serves: 4

4 6-oz sea bass fillets with skin
2 T. macadamia nut oil
½ t. fresh rosemary leaves, coarsely chopped
½ t. fresh thyme leaves
Macadamia nut oil, for brushing

1 T. high-quality liquid fish oil (optional)
Fresh ground black pepper, to taste

Rub the skinless sides of the fillets with 1 T. of the macadamia nut oil. Sprinkle with the herbs and season with some black pepper. Sandwich the fillets together (2 groups of 2 fillets), skin side outward and loosely tie with kitchen string. Rub the skin sides with the remaining macadamia nut oil and season with some black pepper.

Brush the grill surface with some macadamia nut oil then bring the grill to a moderate-low heat. Grill the fish until just cooked through and the skin is browned and crisp, about 12 minutes per side. Remove the kitchen string, transfer one sea bass fillet to the center of each plate, drizzle with fish oil, season with some black pepper and serve immediately. Great with Californian, Australian, New Zealand or Chilean Sauvignon Blanc, Sancerre or dry white Bordeaux.

PER SERVING
Calories: 234
Protein (grams): 36
Fat: 10
Carbohydrates: 0
Fiber: 0

Seared Sea Scallops with Fennel-Orange Sauce

Serves: 4

1 T. extra-virgin olive oil
1 large fennel bulb, cored and cut lengthwise into ¾ inch long strips
1 medium yellow onion, peeled and thinly sliced
2 garlic cloves, peeled and minced
¼ t. fennel seeds

1 cup Vegetable Stock (see above recipe)
½ T. Pernod
1 small seedless orange
1 celery stalk, peeled and cut into ¾ inch long strips
½ small red onion, peeled and cut into ¾ inch long strips
½ T. extra-virgin olive oil
½ t. apple cider vinegar
1 T. macadamia nut oil
12 large sea scallops
½ T. fresh snipped chives
1 T. high-quality liquid fish oil (optional)
Fresh ground black pepper, to taste

Melt the olive oil in a large saucepan. Add all but ½ cup of the fennel as well as the yellow onion, garlic and fennel seeds. Sauté over moderate-low heat until the fennel is crisp-tender, about 20 minutes. Add the vegetable stock, bring to a simmer, cover and cook over low heat until all the vegetables have softened, about 20 minutes more. Let cool then purée in batches in a food processor or blender. Strain into a small saucepan, add the Pernod, season with some black pepper and keep warm.

Peel the orange and remove all the orange sections. Add the celery, red onion, macadamia nut oil, apple cider vinegar and reserved ½ cup of fennel, toss and season with some black pepper. Add to the fennel broth.

In a large skillet, heat the macadamia nut oil until shimmering. Season the scallops with some black pepper, then add to the skillet, cooking over moderate-high heat until browned, about 2 minutes per side. Place 3 scallops in the center of each plate, spoon some fennel-orange sauce on top, garnish with the chives, drizzle with fish oil, season with some black pepper then serve immediately. Great with Californian, Australian, New Zealand or Chilean Sauvignon Blanc, Sancerre or dry white Bordeaux.

PER SERVING
Calories: 406

Protein (grams): 19
Fat: 22
Carbohydrates: 31
Fiber: 7

♟

Grilled Shrimp with Basil-Mint Purée

Serves: 4

¼ cup raw pistachios
¾ cup fresh basil leaves, coarsely chopped
¼ cup fresh mint leaves, coarsely chopped
1 T. fresh lime juice
1 T. rice vinegar
¼ t. dry mustard
¼ t. ground cayenne pepper
¼ cup extra-virgin olive oil
4 1-inch ice cubes
Macadamia nut oil, for brushing
2 pounds large shrimp, shelled and deveined, tails left on
1 T. high-quality liquid fish oil (optional)
Fresh ground black pepper, to taste

Preheat the oven to 400°F. Spread the pistachios on a baking sheet and toast for about 5 minutes, or until fragrant. Let cool then coarsely chop.

In a food processor, combine the chopped pistachios with the basil, mint, lime juice, cayenne pepper and olive oil until puréed. Add the ice cubes and blend until sauce is very smooth. Scrape into small bowl and season with some black pepper.

Brush the grill surface with some macadamia nut oil then bring the grill to a medium-high heat. Brush the shrimp with macadamia nut oil and season with some black pepper. Grill for about 2 minutes per side until lightly charred and just cooked through.

Transfer the shrimp onto the center of each plate, spoon some basil-mint purée on top, drizzle with fish oil, season with some black pepper and serve immediately. Great with Californian, Australian, New Zealand or Chilean Sauvignon Blanc, Sancerre or dry white Bordeaux.

PER SERVING
Calories: 302
Protein (grams): 21
Fat: 22
Carbohydrates: 5
Fiber: 5

♟

Spicy Shrimp and Calamari Sauté

Serves: 4

3 garlic cloves, peeled and minced
½ t. ground coriander
½ t. ground cardamom
¼ t. hot paprika
½ pound medium shrimp, shelled, deveined and cut into medium dice
½ pound cleaned squid, bodies cut into 1/4-inch rings and tentacles halved
4 T. extra-virgin olive oil (or 2 T. olive oil and 2 T. macadamia nut oil)
1 small onion, peeled and cut into medium dice
1 Serrano pepper, seeded and finely chopped
Juice and finely grated zest of 1 small lemon
1 T. fresh mint leaves, coarsely chopped
1 T. high-quality liquid fish oil (optional)
Fresh ground black pepper, to taste

In a small bowl, combine the garlic, coriander, cardamom and paprika. Place the shrimp and squid in separate bowls and season each with equal parts of the spice mixture. Add 1 T. of olive oil to each bowl and toss well.

Heat the remaining 2 T. of olive oil in a large heavy skillet. Add the onion and Serrano pepper and cook over moderate heat until starting to brown, about 8 minutes. Transfer the solids to a large bowl using a slotted spoon and mix in the lemon juice, lemon zest and mint leaves.

Reheat the oil in the skillet. Add the shrimp and stir-fry over high heat for about 2 minutes. Transfer the shrimp to the large bowl using a slotted spoon. Add the squid to the hot skillet and stir-fry for about 2 minutes. Transfer the contents of the skillet to the large bowl and toss well.

Place an equal amount of the sauté onto the center of each plate. Drizzle with fish oil, season with the black pepper and serve immediately. Great with German or Alsatian Riesling or Alsatian Pinot Gris or Gewürtztraminer.

PER SERVING
Calories: 373
Protein (grams): 27
Fat: 24
Carbohydrates: 10
Fiber: 2

Deep-Sautéed Tuna with Ginger-Scallion Sauce

Serves: 4

1½ cups macadamia nut oil

1½ lbs. fresh yellowfin tuna steaks (at least 1 inch thick), cut into 8 equal portions
1½ t. fresh ginger, peeled and minced
10 large scallions, thinly sliced
3 T. balsamic vinegar
2. T. low-sodium soy sauce
1 T. ketchup
1 T. extra-virgin olive oil
1 T. high-quality liquid fish oil (optional)
Fresh ground black pepper, to taste

In a medium saucepan, heat the macadamia nut oil until a piece of scallion sizzles in it. Season the tuna steaks with some black pepper and carefully add to the saucepan. The fish should be completely immersed in oil. Reduce the heat to look and cook for about 5 minutes (medium rare). Transfer to a plate and cover with foil to keep warm.

In a small saucepan, reheat 3 T. of the tuna cooking oil over low hear. Add the scallions and ginger and cook for about 10 minutes, until the scallions become tender. Add the balsamic vinegar, soy sauce and ketchup and simmer for 2 more minutes. Remove from the heat, blend in the olive oil and season with some black pepper.

Transfer 2 tuna pieces onto the center of each plate. Spread some scallions and sauce on top, drizzle with fish oil, season with some black pepper and serve immediately. Great with German or Alsatian Riesling or Alsatian Pinot Gris or Gewürtztraminer.

PER SERVING
Calories: 421
Protein (grams): 28
Fat: 25
Carbohydrates: 21
Fiber: 3

♟

Paprika-Coated Trout with Cilantro-Almond Sauce

Serves: 4

½ cup raw almonds
1 large egg
1 t. macadamia nut oil
¼ cup whole wheat flour
1 t. sweet paprika
1 t. hot paprika
4 6-oz fresh mountain trout fillets, skin removed, about ¾ inch thick
1½ cups packed fresh cilantro leaves and tender stems
3 T. fresh lemon juice
¼ cup plus 1 T. extra-virgin olive oil
1 T. high-quality liquid fish oil (optional)
Fresh ground black pepper, to taste

Preheat the oven to 400°F. Toast the almonds on a small baking plate for about 5 minutes, or until fragrant. In a small bowl, beat the egg with the macadamia nut oil. On a plate, combine the flour with the sweet paprika and half of the hot paprika.

Dip each fish fillet into the beaten egg, letting any excess drip off. Coat the fillets with the seasoned flour, place on wire rack set over baking sheet and refrigerate for about 20 minutes, until the coating has set.

Meanwhile, in a food processor, combine the cilantro, lemon juice, almonds and the remaining hot paprika until coarsely chopped. With the machine running, gradually drizzle in ¼ cup of the olive oil and mix until well blended.

Heat the remaining olive oil in a large skillet. Add the fish and sauté over moderate-high heat until the coating is crisp and the fish is cooked through, about 3 minutes per side.

Transfer 1 fillet onto the center of each plate, spoon some sauce over top, drizzle with fish oil, season with the black pepper and serve immediately. Great with Californian or Australian Chardonnay or white Burgundy.

PER SERVING
Calories: 495
Protein (grams): 30
Fat: 31
Carbohydrates: 15
Fiber: 4

♟

Lobster with Burgundy Sauce

Serves: 4

Four 1¼ lb. live lobsters
1 T. extra-virgin olive oil
1 large shallot, peeled and finely chopped
2 large garlic cloves, peeled and finely chopped
1 cup Pinot Noir (Californian, Oregonian or French)
1 cup Demi-Glace (see above recipe)
2 T. port (Ruby or Late-Bottled Vintage)
1 T. macadamia nut oil
2 vanilla beans, split lengthwise, seeds scraped (optional)
1 T. high-quality liquid fish oil (optional)
Fresh ground black pepper, to taste

Fill the sink with ice water. Fill a large stockpot 1/3 full with water and bring to a boil. Add the lobsters head first, cover and steam for about

5 minutes. Using tongs, turn the lobsters over and steam for another 5 minutes, until the shells are bright red. Using tongs, transfer the lobsters to the ice water.

Drain the lobsters and pat dry. Crack the shells and remove the meat from the claws and tails, slitting the tails to remove the intestinal vein. Reserve the meat in a small bowl, cutting the tails crosswise into medallions. Using sturdy kitchen shears, cut the lobster shells into 2-inch pieces.

Meanwhile, heat the olive oil in a large saucepan and add the shallot, cooking over moderate heat until just starting to brown, about 3 minutes. Add the garlic and cook for another 2 minutes.

Add the lobster shells and cook for another 8 minutes. Add the red wine and cook for another 10 minutes. Add the Demi-Glace and cook for another 5 minutes. Strain the sauce through a fine-mesh sieve into a medium saucepan, pressing on the solids to remove as much liquid as possible. Add the port, season with some black pepper and simmer over moderate-low heat for 5 minutes. Cover the sauce, remove from the heat and keep warm. In a small bowl, stir the vanilla seeds into the liquid fish oil.

In a large skillet, heat the macadamia nut oil and add the reserved lobster meat, cooking over moderate-low heat for about 4 minutes, until just warmed through. Transfer equal amounts of lobster meat onto the center of each plate. Spoon the sauce around the lobster, dot the plates with the vanilla oil, season with some black pepper and serve immediately. Great with Californian or Oregonian Pinot Noir or red Burgundy.

PER SERVING
Calories: 394
Protein (grams): 35
Fat: 22
Carbohydrates: 14
Fiber: 2

Part VI. Meat
(Serve all Meat Entrées with Steamed/Sautéed Vegetables
or Small Green Salad and ½ Baked Sweet Potato or 1 Cup of
either Wild Rice or Whole Wheat Pasta)

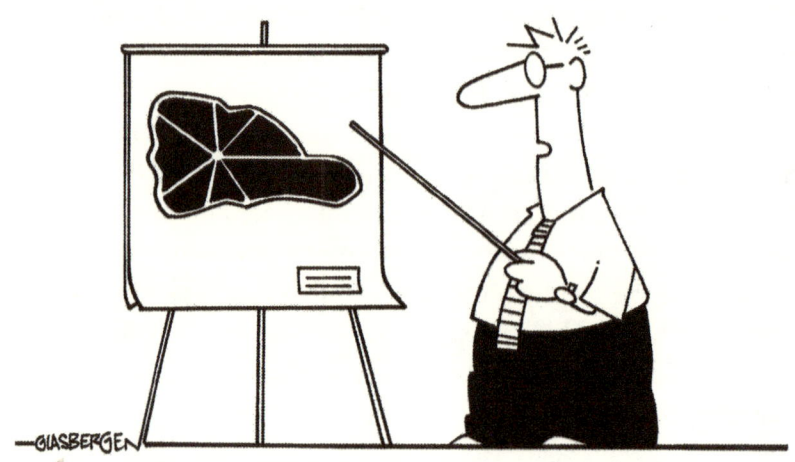

Copyright 2004 by Randy Glasbergen.
www.glasbergen.com

"At the request of those who are following a low-carb diet,
my pie chart has been replaced by a steak chart."

Grilled Beef Tenderloin with Shiraz Sauce

Serves: 4

1 bottle full-bodied Australian Shiraz (or Californian Syrah or Côte du Rhône)
2 shallots, peeled and sliced
1 cup Demi-Glace (see above recipe)
2 T. macadamia nut oil

2 T. HAPI spice mixture (see above recipe)
2 whole cloves, ground
2 allspice berries, ground
1 cup mixed fresh herb leaves (basil, mint and tarragon), cut into thin strips
2 T. white truffle oil
1 T. sherry wine vinegar
4 6-oz. beef tenderloin fillets (center-cut), trimmed of all visible fat
1 T. extra-virgin olive oil
1 T. port (Ruby or Late-Bottled Vintage)
Fresh ground black pepper, to taste
Macadamia nut oil, for brushing

Place Shiraz and shallots in medium pot and bring to a boil over medium-high heat. Cook until reduced to about ¼ cup then strain into clean saucepan and add the Demi-Glace. Keep warm. In a small bowl, blend the 2 T. macadamia nut oil with the HAPI spice mixture, ground cloves and ground allspice berries. Brush this blend onto both flat surfaces of the tenderloin fillets. In another small bowl, whisk the truffle oil and sherry vinegar. Toss in the chopped herb leaves then season with some black pepper.

Brush the grill surface with some of the extra macadamia nut oil then bring the grill to a medium-high heat. Grill the fillets about 5–7 minutes each side until an instead-read thermometer inserted into the center of each fillet reads 125°F (medium rare). Transfer to a clean surface and let cool for about 5 minutes. Return the sauce to a simmer and blend in the olive oil and port. Transfer 1 fillet onto the center of each plate, cover with some sauce, top with a large dollop of the herb salad, season with some black pepper and serve immediately. Great with Hermitage, Cornas or Côte Rôtie.

PER SERVING
Calories: 506
Protein (grams): 27

Fat: 31
Carbohydrates: 23
Fiber: 5

ஃ

Seared Flank Steak with Salsa Verde

Serves: 4

½ cup packed fresh flat-leaf parsley leaves and tender stems
¼ cup packed chopped fresh chives
2 garlic cloves, peeled and minced
6 anchovy fillets (packed in olive oil)
2 T. drained capers
1 t. red wine vinegar
½ cup extra-virgin olive oil
1 T. macadamia nut oil
1 T. HAPI spice mixture (see above recipe)
1 lb. flank steak
Fresh ground black pepper, to taste

In a food processor, pulse the parsley, chives, garlic, anchovies, capers and vinegar until coarsely chopped. With the machine running, drizzle in the olive oil and mix until just blended.

In a large skillet, heat the macadamia nut oil until almost smoking. Season the steak with 1 T. HAPI spice mixture and some black pepper then add to the skillet. Cook over moderately-high heat until well seared outside but still pink inside, about 5 minutes per side (medium-rare). Transfer to a cutting surface and let cool for about 5 minutes. Carve across the grain into thin slices, place an equal amount onto the center of each plate, spoon some salsa verde over top, season with the black pepper and serve immediately. Great with Californian Zinfandel, Australian Shiraz, Gigondas or Chateâuneuf-du-Pape.

PER SERVING
Calories: 308
Protein (grams): 28
Fat: 20
Carbohydrates: 14
Fiber: 3

♟

Pan-Roasted Pork Tenderloin with Porcini, Sun-Dried Tomatoes and Balsamic Sauce

Serves: 4

1 cup Roasted Vegetable Stock (see above recipe)
1 oz package of dried porcini mushrooms
¼ cup sun-dried tomatoes (packed in extra-virgin olive oil), coarsely chopped
3 T. extra-virgin olive oil
1 cup balsamic vinegar
½ cup Demi-Glace (see above recipe)
2 T. HAPI spice mixture (see above recipe)
1 whole clove, ground
1 allspice berry, ground
3 dried porcini mushroom slices, ground
¼ cup macadamia nut oil
1½ lb. boneless pork tenderloin, trimmed of all fat
1 T. extra-virgin olive oil
1 T. Madeira (or dry Sherry)
Fresh ground black pepper, to taste

Preheat oven to 400°F. Place vegetable stock in medium pot, bring just a boil, remove from the heat, mix in the package of dried porcini mushrooms, cover and let sit for about 30 minutes. Strain into a clean pot and keep warm. Rinse the reconstituted mushrooms several times in fresh water to remove all grit then place between some paper towels and press firmly to remove all moisture.

Heat 2 T. of the olive oil in a medium saucepan over medium-high heat then add the chopped sun-dried tomatoes and reconstituted mushrooms. Sauté until the vegetables just start to brown (about 4 minutes) then add the porcini stock and the balsamic vinegar. Cook until the liquid has been reduced to about ½ cup then lower the heat, mix in the Demi-Glace and keep warm.

Meanwhile, in a small bowl, blend 2 T. of the macadamia nut oil with the HAPI spice mixture, ground clove, ground allspice and ground porcini. Brush this blend all over the pork tenderloin surface and season with some black pepper.

In a large skillet, heat the remaining 2 T. of macadamia nut oil until almost smoking. Add the pork tenderloin to the skillet and sear each side until well-browned, about 2 minutes per side. Place the skillet into the oven and roast for about 8–10 minutes, until a thermometer inserted into the center reads 150°F (medium). Transfer to a cutting surface and let cool for about 5 minutes.

Return the sauce to a simmer and blend in the remaining 1 T. of olive oil and the Madeira. Cut the tenderloin into 8 slices then place 2 of them onto the center of each plate. Cover with some sauce, season with some black pepper and serve immediately. Great with Amarone, Barolo or Barbaresco.

PER SERVING
Calories: 492
Protein (grams): 36
Fat: 32
Carbohydrates: 15
Fiber: 3

Ⱥ

Braised Lamb Shanks with Bell Peppers and Garlic

Serves: 4

4 lamb shanks (about 1 lb. each)
1 T. HAPI spice mixture (see above recipe)
1 T. ground thyme
36 whole garlic gloves, 24 peeled and 12 unpeeled
6 bay leaves
6 fresh thyme sprigs plus 1 T. fresh thyme leaves
4 cups Roasted Vegetable Stock (see above recipe)
1 large red bell pepper, cored, halved and cut into ¼ inch strips
1 large yell bell pepper, cored, halved and cut into ¼ inch strips
1 T. extra-virgin olive oil
Fresh ground black pepper, to taste

Preheat the oven to 300°F. Season the lamb shanks with the HAPI spice mixture, ground thyme and some black pepper. In a large cast-iron pot large enough to contain all the shanks, combine the lamb shanks with the unpeeled garlic cloves, bay leaves and thyme sprigs. Cook over moderate heat, turning every 5 minutes until well browned all over, about 15 minutes. Cover the pot, place in the oven and roast for 2 hours, until very tender, turning every 20 minutes. Remove from the oven and let stand, covered, for about 20 minutes.

Remove the lamb shanks and set aside on a clean surface. Add the stock to the pot, bring to a boil over high heat (scraping up any browned bits on the bottom) and reduce to 2 cups, about 10 minutes.

Strain the stock and return to the pot. Add the peeled garlic cloves and simmer over medium-low heat until tender, about 20 minutes. Return the shanks to the pot along with the bell peppers and thyme leaves. Cover and simmer until the peppers become tender, about 10 minutes.

Transfer 1 lamb shank onto the center of each plate. Blend the olive oil into the sauce. Cover each shank with some sauce, season with some black pepper then serve immediately. Great with Californian or Oregonian Pinot Noir or red Burgundy.

PER SERVING
Calories: 279
Protein (grams): 26
Fat: 11
Carbohydrates: 19
Fiber: 6

Spicy Chicken A' La Orange

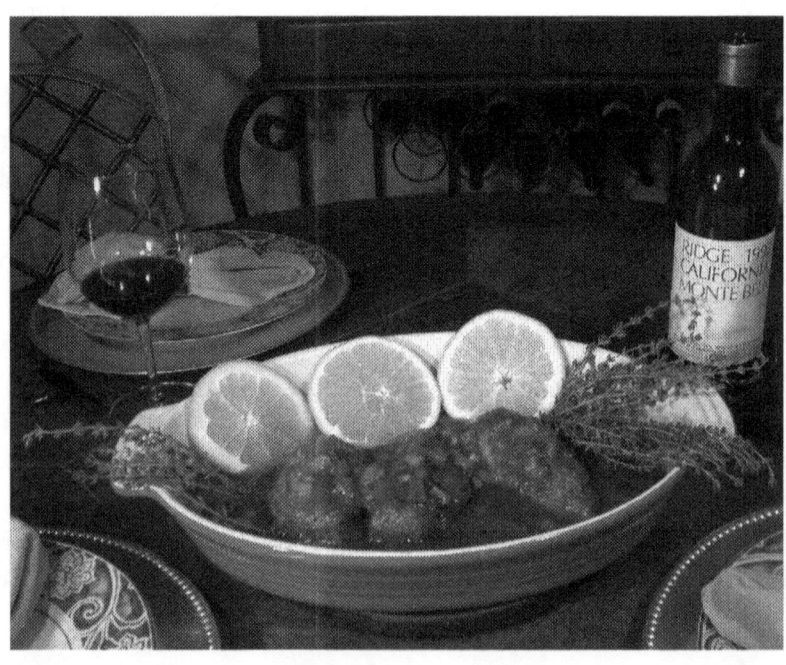

Serves: 4

4 6-oz chicken breasts, boneless, skinless
½ cup whole wheat flour
2 T. HAPI spice mixture (see above recipe)
½ T. ground cayenne pepper
½ T. ground thyme
¼ cup macadamia nut oil
1 cup fresh orange juice, strained
½ cup chili sauce
2 T. low-sodium soy sauce
2 T. blackstrap molasses
1 T. Dijon mustard
1 yellow bell pepper, cored, cut into large dice
1 red bell pepper, cored, cut into large dice
4 garlic cloves, minced
1 T. extra-virgin olive oil
1 T. Grand Marnier (or other orange-flavored brandy)
Fresh ground black pepper, to taste

Preheat the oven to 350°F. On a plate, combine the whole wheat flour with the HAPI spice mixture, cayenne pepper and thyme. Dredge the chicken breasts in the seasoned flour, shaking off any excess then season with some black pepper. In a medium bowl, whisk together the orange juice, chili sauce, soy sauce, molasses and mustard.

In a large skillet, heat the macadamia nut oil and add the chicken breasts, cooking over moderate-high heat for about 2 minutes per side. Transfer the chicken breasts to a casserole. Add the bell peppers and garlic and sauté for about 3 minutes. Add the contents of the medium bowl and simmer for another 3 minutes. Pour sauce over the chicken breasts in the casserole, cover then bake for about 50–55 minutes until quite tender. Remove from the oven, blend in the olive oil and Grand Marnier and let stand for 5 minutes.

Transfer 1 chicken breast onto the center of each plate. Cover with some sauce, season with some black pepper then serve immediately. Great with Californian, Washingtonian, Chilean or Australian Cabernet Sauvignon or red Bordeaux.

PER SERVING
Calories: 508
Protein (grams): 51
Fat: 20
Carbohydrates: 31
Fiber: 8

♙

Rustic Frittata with Garlic, Sun-Dried Tomatoes and Wild Mushrooms

Serves: 4

1½ cups plain Egg Beaters
½ cup grated imported Parmigiano-Reggiano cheese
¼ cup fresh basil leaves, coarsely chopped
2 T. extra-virgin olive oil (or 1 T. olive oil and 1 T. macadamia nut oil)
1 small yellow onion, peeled and cut into medium dice
½ head garlic, separated into cloves (about 12), peeled and cut in half lengthwise
½ cup shitake mushrooms, stemmed and caps thickly sliced
¼ cup sun-dried tomatoes (packed in extra-virgin olive oil), coarsely chopped
1 T. oil from jar of sun-dried tomatoes
1 T. white truffle oil
Fresh ground black pepper, to taste

In a large bowl, whisk the Egg Beaters and cheese together until well blended then mix in the basil. Set aside.

In a medium ovenproof skillet, heat the olive oil and add the onion and garlic, cooking over moderate heat until starting to brown, about 5 minutes. Add the mushrooms and sun-dried tomatoes, season with some black pepper and cook for another 5 minutes. Transfer the contents of the skillet into the large bowl and mix together.

Heat the sun-dried tomato oil in the same medium skillet then add the contents of the large bowl, spreading the vegetables evenly across the surface of the skillet. Cook over medium-low heat until the bottom is set, about 10 minutes. Place the skillet under the broiler for about 2 minutes, until cooked through. Brush the truffle oil evenly over the surface of the frittata, season with some black pepper, cut into 4 wedges and place 1 wedge onto the center of each plate. Serve immediately. Great with Mimosa using Moscato d' Asti in place of Champagne.

PER SERVING
Calories: 335
Protein (grams): 19
Fat: 23
Carbohydrates: 13
Fiber: 3

Chapter Nine
A Day on the 'HAPI Heart Diet'

Copyright 2002 by Randy Glasbergen.   www.glasbergen.com

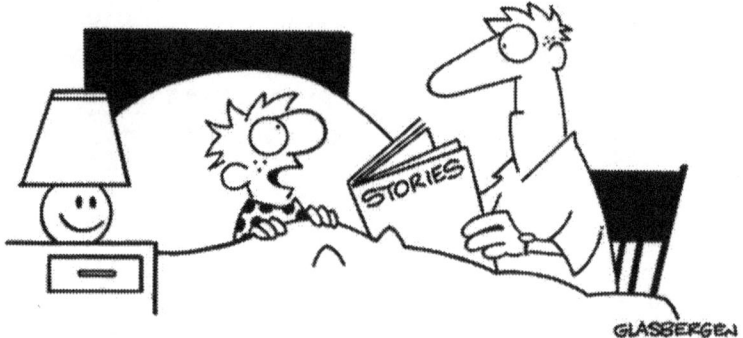

**"Snow White was poisoned by an apple,
Jack found a giant in his beanstalk, and look
what happened to Alice when she ate the mushroom!
And you wonder why I won't eat fruit and vegetables!?"**

I'm a 5'9" man weighing between 165 and 175 pounds. My IBW would be right around 160 (± 16) pounds. I walk about 6000–7500 steps per day (not including exercise). My total daily calories should therefore be around 1900–2300 (not including post-workout meals). The following might be a typical day for me on the HAPI Heart Diet.

Two 8-oz glasses of water upon awakening

Breakfast:
Cup of green tea
2 Fiber-Choice sugar-free wafers (8 grams of soluble fiber)
½ cup sliced cremini mushrooms
¼ cup yellow onion, peeled and cut into medium dice
2 T. carrot, peeled and cut into medium dice
2 T. celery stalk, cut into medium dice
2 T. macadamia nut oil (to sauté the above vegetables)
¼ cup plain Egg Beaters, scrambled
2 T. fresh blueberries

Two 8-oz glasses of water and one fresh raw apple right before exercise

Exercise (375 calories expended):
30 minutes on treadmill
5 minutes of stretching
15 minutes of lifting weights

One 8-oz glass of water every 15 minutes of exercise and another 8-oz glass of water after finishing exercise

Post-Workout Meal (within 30 minutes of finishing exercise):
1 cup non-fat plain yogurt
2 T. non-fat plain cottage cheese, soaked in water to remove salt
1 cup fresh strawberries, sliced

One 8-oz glass of water before snack

Mid-Morning Snack:
Cup of green tea (optional)
3 large celery stalks
1 large carrot, peeled

½ cup fresh raw broccoli flowerets
¼ cup natural almond butter

One 8-oz glass of water before lunch

Lunch:
Cup of green tea
2 Fiber-Choice sugar-free wafers
1 cup mixed baby greens, washed
¼ cup fresh grape tomatoes, sliced in half
½ avocado, sliced
Vinaigrette made from 1 T. hazelnut oil and ½ T. sherry wine vinegar
2 T. non-fat plain cottage cheese, soaked in water to remove salt
½ oz raw almonds

One 8-oz glass of water before snack

Mid-Afternoon Snack:
Cup of green tea (optional)
1 cup mixed canned black beans, red kidney beans and garbanzo beans, soaked and rinsed in water very well to remove salt
Vinaigrette made from 1 T. extra-virgin olive oil and ½ T. balsamic vinegar
2 T. non-fat plain cottage cheese, soaked in water to remove salt
2 T. fresh blackberries

One 8-oz glass of water before dinner

Dinner:
1–2 glasses of red wine (e.g. Californian or Oregonian Pinot Noir) or white wine (e.g. German or Alsatian Riesling)
2 Fiber-Choice sugar-free wafers
½ cup mixed baby greens, washed
2 T. fresh grape tomatoes, sliced in half

2 T. red bell pepper, cut into medium dice
Vinaigrette made from 1 T. extra-virgin olive oil and ½ T. fresh lemon juice
1 T. non-fat plain cottage cheese, soaked in water to remove salt
1 T. fresh blueberries
½ oz raw pecans
¼ cup fresh steamed broccoli flowerets
½ baked sweet potato
Pan-Roasted Salmon with Sun-Dried Tomato-Kalamata Sauce (see above recipe)

Two 8-oz glasses of water and one fresh raw pear right before exercise

Exercise (155 calories expended):
15 minutes on exercise bike
5 minutes of stretching

One 8-oz glass of water after finishing exercise

Post-Workout Evening Meal (within 30 minutes of finishing exercise):
1 cup green tea (optional)
1 cup All-Bran cereal, plain
½ cup skim milk
¼ cup fresh raspberries

One 8-oz glass of water before going to bed

Calories: 2243 (+531 pre/post-exercise)
Protein (grams): 110 (+35) (21% calories)
Fat: 139 (+3) (48%)
TFA: 0
ω-6 PUFA: 17 (5%)
SFA: 16 (+1) (5%)
Cholesterol (mg): 122 (+15)
ω-3 PUFA (grams): 3
ω-9 MUFA: 113 (+2) (37%)
Carbohydrates: 129 (+91) (31%)
Fiber: 55 (+18)
Sodium (mg): 1153 (+390)

Chapter Ten
Optimal Medical Diagnosis and Treatment of Dyslipoproteinemia

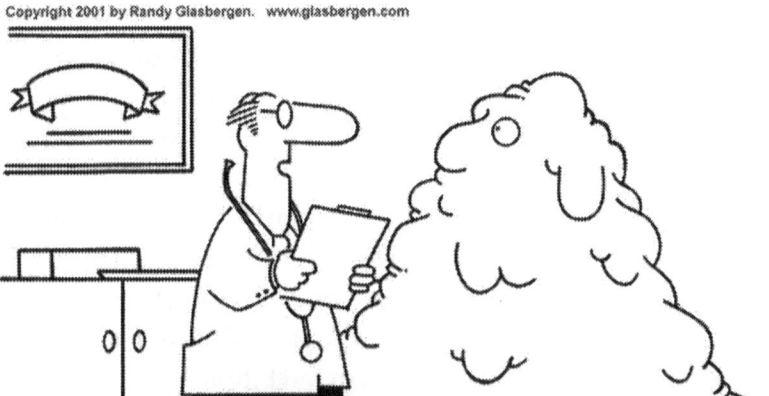

Copyright 2001 by Randy Glasbergen. www.glasbergen.com

"You haven't been taking your cholesterol medication, have you Mr. Grosshart?"

In this chapter (intended mainly for physicians), we will: 1) describe the main mechanisms of action of the various lipid-modifying pharmaceuticals; and 2) put all the principles of this book together in the analysis of an actual patient case.

Part I. Lipid-Modifying Drugs

In my opinion, pharmaceutical agents for dyslipoproteinemia should only be used when nutritional and other such lifestyle modalities have proven ineffective. In a patient with known CHD and/or type II DM, I usually recommend both drastic lifestyle changes as well as pharmaceutical therapy from the onset. If the patient actually makes the necessary lifestyle changes, the patient and I may later decide to taper off some of the medications and this typically will work to some extent. On the other hand, if I have a patient with high risk for later CHD and/or type II DM (but no actual evidence of these disease states at present), I usually promote appropriate lifestyle changes for around six months and only consider adding medications if things don't work out during that time period. For people with lower risk of future CHD and/or type II DM, I typically recommend necessary dietary and exercise modalities and only add medications as a 'last resort' after 12 months or so.

The medications used for dyslipoproteinemia include Statins (Crestor, Lescol, Lipitor, Mevacor, Pravachol, Zocor), cholesterol absorption inhibitors (CAI—Zetia), combination Statin+CAI (Vytorin), bile acid sequestrants (BAS—Questran, Welchol), prescription Niacin (Niaspan), combination Statin+Niacin (Advicor), Fibrates (Lopid, Tricor), Glitazones (Actos, Avandia) and prescription fish oils (Omacor).

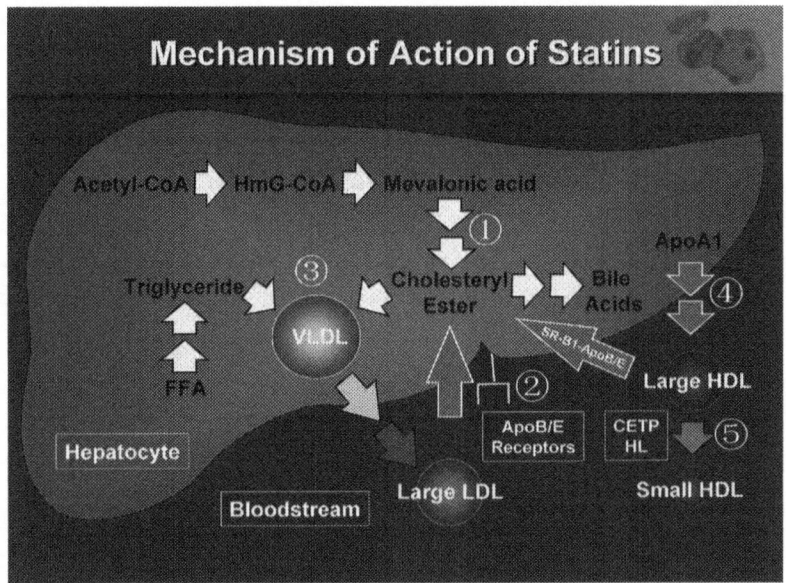

Image 28: Mechanism Of Action of Statins

Statins work by multiple mechanisms (see Image 28 above). 1) Statins block the hepatic enzyme HmG-CoA reductase with which the liver manufactures CE. A reliable bloodstream marker of this reduction in hepatic CE production would be reduced serum lathosterol levels. The liver normally uses CE to form bile acids to assist digestion as well as VLDL particles to transport CE, TG, phospholipid (PL) and Coenzyme Q10 (CoQ10) to the various tissues of the body. 2) The diminished levels of CE in the hepatocyte cause it to up-regulate ApoB/E receptors which remove large (primarily), CE-rich LDL particles from the bloodstream. 3) When hepatic CE levels are diminished, the hepatocyte also decreases its production and secretion of VLDL particles. 4) Statins increase the production of ApoA1 and thus HDL particles to some extent (some Statins more than others). 5) Statins also weakly inhibit cholesteryl ester transport protein (CETP) and hepatic lipase (HL) and thus tend to increase HDL particle size (and LDL particle size). By the way, since Statins block the production of CoQ10 (normally made whenever CE is made), some feel that anyone taking a Statin should also take a CoQ10 supplement. Statins should not be used in individuals with any ongoing liver problems but (despite what the TV ads suggest) are probably quite safe in anyone with a 'normal' liver. In fact, in my experience, abnormal liver tests in individuals taking Statins usually represent fatty liver and what is really required is weight loss and dietary changes. But anyone taking a Statin who notices new muscle tenderness, weakness or swelling should stop the medication and notify their doctor immediately.

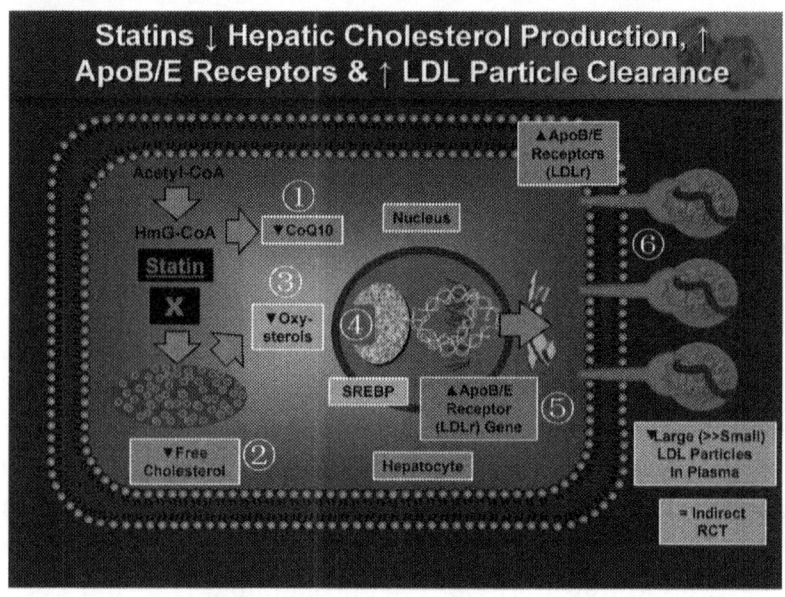

Image 29: Statins ↓ Hepatic Cholesterol Production, ↑ ApoB/E Receptors & ↑ LDL Particle Clearance

Statins diminish intra-hepatic free cholesterol (FC) levels to increase the clearance of mainly large LDL particles, thus enhancing the 'benign' CE circuit (see Image 29 above). 1) Through the inhibition of HmG-CoA reductase, CoQ10 production is decreased as mentioned above. 2) FC levels within the hepatocyte are likewise reduced. 3) The resultant decrease in oxysterols sends a signal to the nucleus of the hepatocyte. 4) Sterol response element binding protein (SREBP) is stimulated and attaches to the ApoB/E receptor gene. 5) Increased amounts of ApoB/E receptors are produced and sent to the surface of the hepatocyte. 6) These ApoB/E receptors recognize mainly large LDL particles and remove them from the circulation.

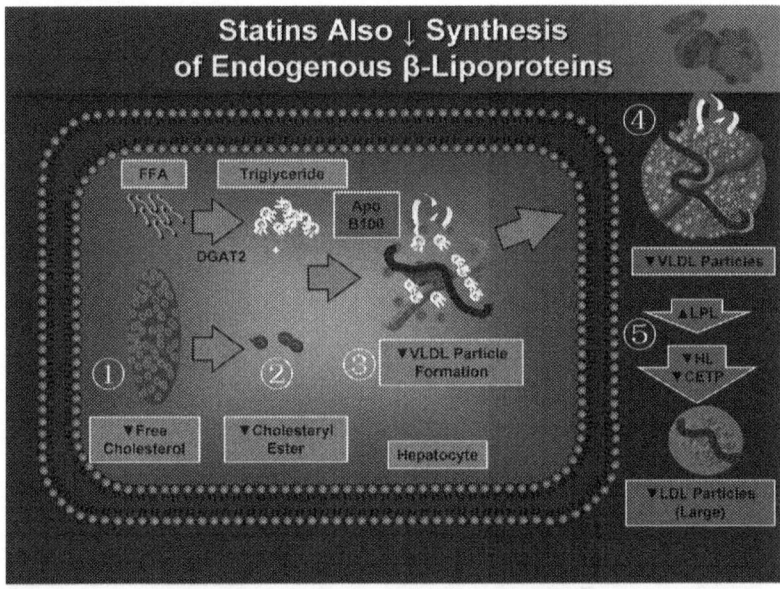

Image 30: Statins Also ↓Synthesis of
Endogenous β-lipoproteins

Statins also decrease the synthesis of endogenous β-lipoproteins (see Image 30 above). 1) FC levels within the hepatocyte are reduced. 2) CE levels are thus decreased. 3) Less VLDL particles are created. 4) Less VLDL particles are secreted into the bloodstream. 5) Decreased amounts of LDL particles in the bloodstream thus result. Since Statins are weak promoters of LPL and inhibitors of HL and CETP, the resultant LDL particles tend to be somewhat larger in size.

Finally, Statins increase the formation of ApoA1 and HDL particles (see Image 31 below). 1) By blocking HmG-CoA reductase, Statins decrease the formation of RhoA Phosphorylase, an enzyme that normally inhibits peroxisome proliferator-activated receptor (PPAR)-α. 2)

PPAR-α can thus be stimulated by its natural ligands. 3) ApoA1 gene expression occurs. 4) Increased amounts of ApoA1 are produced. 5) Increased numbers of nascent HDL particles are secreted into the bloodstream. 6) As Statins are weak CETP and HL inhibitors, the resultant mature HDL particles tend to remain large in size.

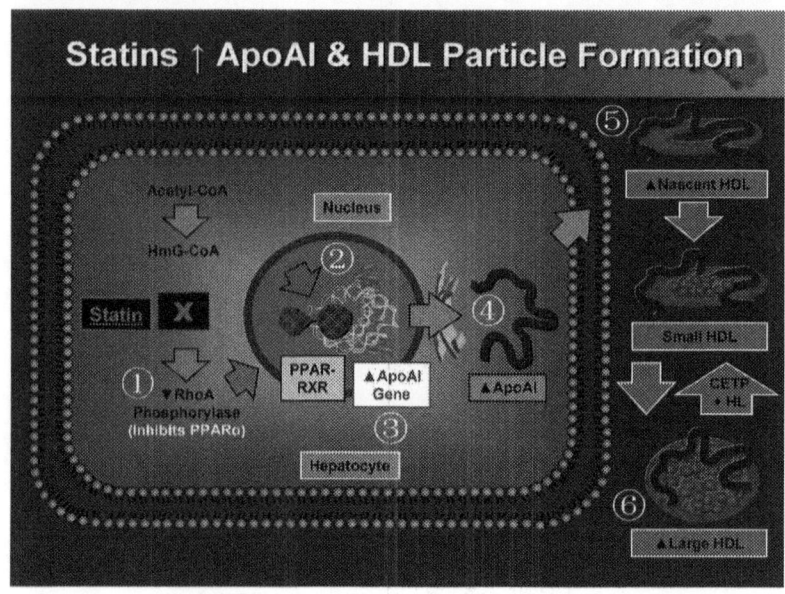

Image 31: Statins ↑ApoA1 & HDL Particle Formation

In the lipid 'shadow' world, Statins decrease LDL-C (removing large, CE-rich LDL particles), decrease TG (reducing VLDL particle production) and increase HDL-C (enhancing HDL particle production and size) (see Image 32 below). But the reason people take Statins is not to make these numbers (whether lipid-based or lipoprotein-based) look 'pretty' on a piece of paper. People take Statins to decrease the future likelihood of heart attacks, strokes and/or premature CV death. However, if you look at the major clinical studies involving many thousands of patients, Statins only prevented 20–30% of major CV events in individuals otherwise predestined to have them. Another way of thinking about these results is that 70–80% of individuals in these trials who were otherwise predestined to have future CV events and took Statins had those CV events anyway.

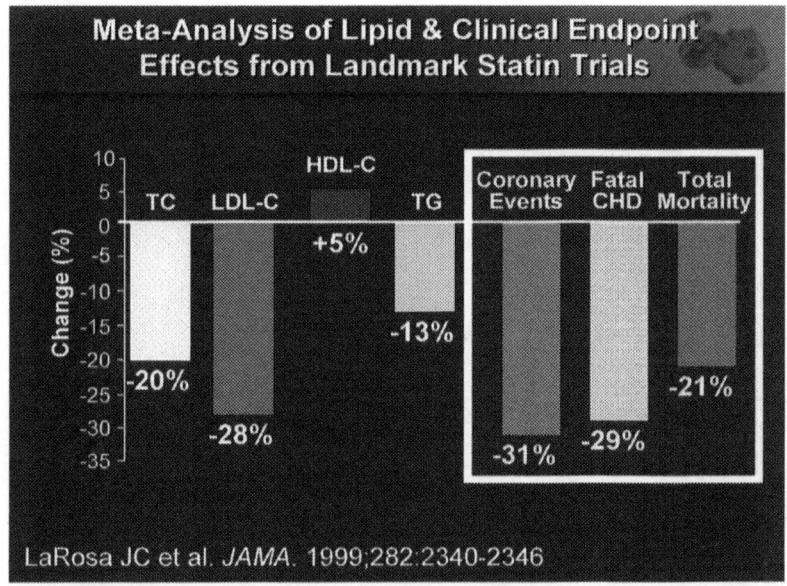

Image 32: Meta-Analysis of Lipid & Clinical Endpoint Effects from Landmark Statin Trials

Another way to decrease FC levels within the hepatocyte is to block cholesterol absorption from the gut (see Image 33 below). 1) Plant stanols (like Benecol) do it by diminishing the FC content in the spherical micelles. 2) BAS (Questran/Welchol) do it by blocking the absorption of bile acids (made from CE) in the last part of the small intestine (ileum). 3) CAI (Zetia) does it by blocking the uptake of FC from the micelles in the first part of the small intestine (duodenum/jejunum).

The most common of the intestinal-acting agents currently used by physicians is Zetia (ezetimibe). Intra-hepatic FC levels are dependent both on the production of cholesterol within hepatocytes as well as the absorption of cholesterol from the gut. Some people are natural 'hyper-absorbers' while others are 'hyper-producers.' Most people are probably a degree of both. Zetia has very few side effects and seems quite safe although people with ongoing liver problems should probably not take it.

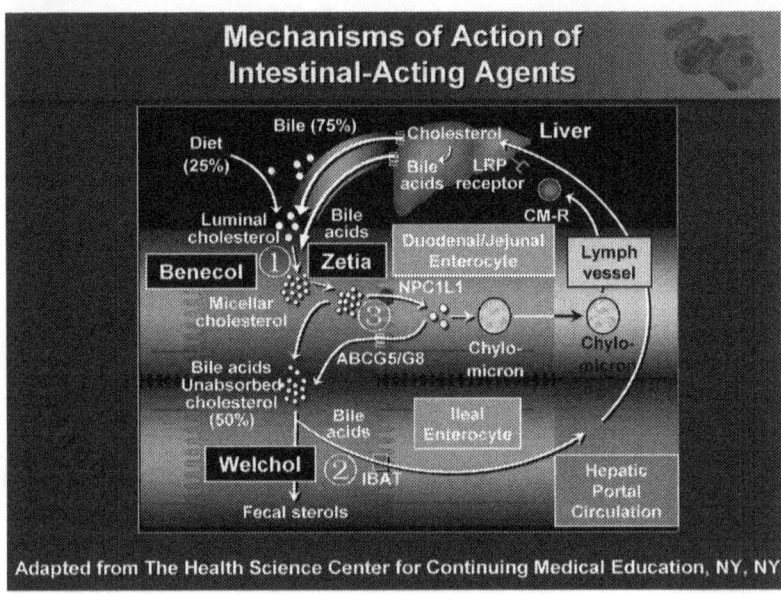

Image 33: Mechanisms of Action of
Intestinal-Acting Agents

There is some evidence demonstrating that patients taking Statins eventually hyper-absorb cholesterol from their gut as an attempt by the body to return to balance. Other sterols that may be even more harmful than cholesterol (sitosterol, campesterol, stigmasterol) may also be absorbed in this situation (see Image 34 below).

Zetia may be useful both as an alternative to Statin therapy for removing primarily large, CE-rich LDL particles from the bloodstream as well as an addition to Statin therapy to enhance LDL particle clearance and potentially prevent the complications of gut cholesterol hyper-absorption (see Image 35 below). A combination Statin + CAI product called Vytorin is now available. 1) Zetia blocks the sterol permease Niemann

Pick C1 Like 1 (NPC1L1) and thus inhibits gut absorption of FC from the micelles. A reliable bloodstream marker of this reduction in gut FC absorption would be reduced serum campesterol levels. 2) Chylomicron and CM-R particles (having less CE in their cores) are secreted into the portal lympatics. 3) Decrease in CM-R particle delivery of CE to the hepatocyte via LDL-related protein (LRP) receptors occurs. 4) The resultant diminished intra-hepatic FC levels lead to increased clearance of large LDL particles and decreased production of VLDL particles. There are currently no published clinical outcome trials involving either Zetia or Benecol but older studies involving BAS showed prevention of 15–20% of otherwise preventable future major CV events.

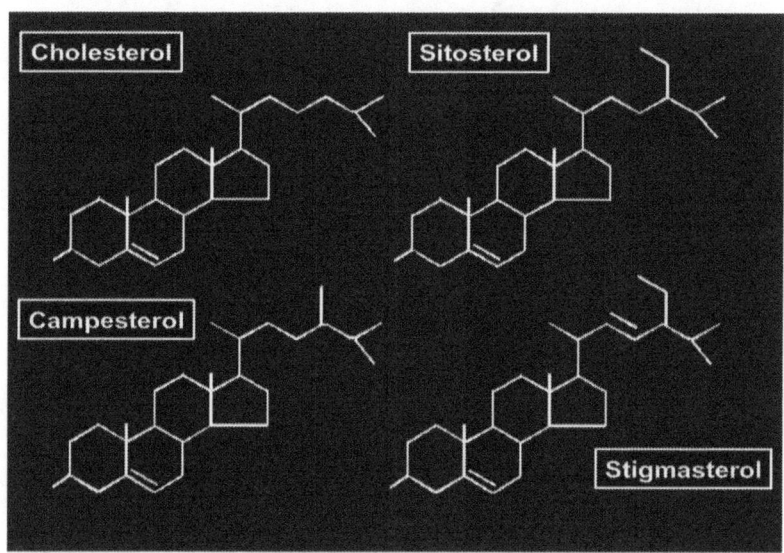

Image 34: Chemical Structures of Cholesterol
and Other Related Sterols

Niacin (vitamin B3) works by multiple mechanisms. First and foremost, Niacin decreases the synthesis of VLDL particles and leads to reduced amounts of LDL particles which tend to be larger (see Image 36 below). 1) Niacin blocks hormone sensitive lipase (HSL) in visceral adipocytes to reduce free fatty acid (FFA) production and secretion.

This leads to diminished intra-hepatic FFA levels. 2) Niacin blocks the conversion of FFA into TG. 3) This causes diminished production of VLDL particles within the hepatocyte. 4) VLDL particle secretion slows and the particles tend to be smaller with less TG in their cores. 5) Niacin also is a potent inhibitor of HL leading to large, CE-rich LDL particles in somewhat reduced concentrations. Niacin should not be taken by individuals with ongoing liver problems or signs of active arterial bleeding. Higher doses of certain forms of dietary supplement Niacin have been shown to cause significant liver inflammation in some individuals.

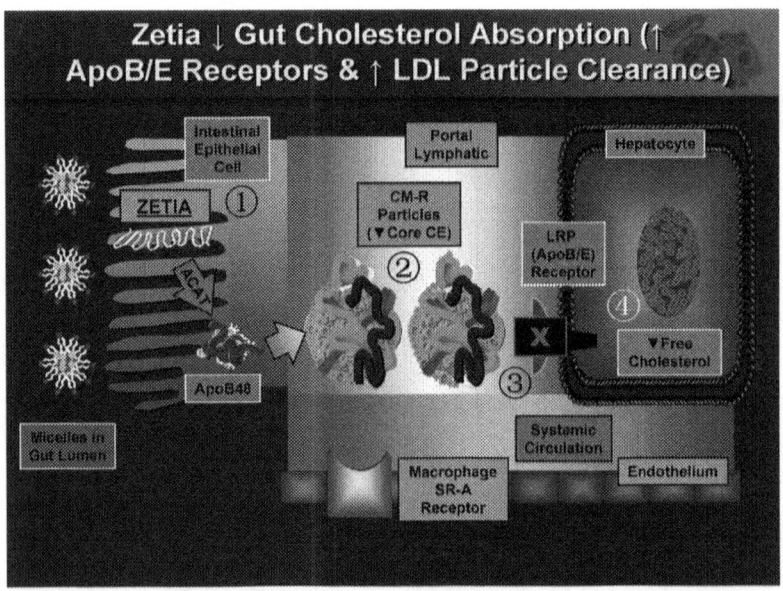

Image 35: Zetia ↓Gut Cholesterol Absorption (↑ApoB/E Receptors & ↑LDL Particle Clearance)

Niacin also has effects upon HDL particle dynamics (see Image 37 below). 1) Large HDL particles can bind via surface ApoA1 to ApoA1, 'holoparticle,' catabolic receptors present on hepatocytes (small HDL particles are not recognized). When large HDL particles bind to these receptors, the entire complex is taken into the hepatocyte and catabolized. 2) Niacin blocks these receptors, thus preventing large HDL particle catabolism (a form of direct reverse cholesterol transport [RCT]). 3) Large HDL particles can also be recognized and de-lipidated by SR-B1 receptors (another form of direct RCT). 4) Large, CE-rich HDL particles can exchange CE for TG with TG-rich β-lipoproteins via CETP. 5) CE can thus be returned to the liver by ApoB/E receptors (indirect RCT). 6) Niacin also blocks HL and the resultant large TG-enriched HDL particles remain in circulation—no longer capable of conversion to small HDL particles, indirect RCT or most forms of direct RCT.

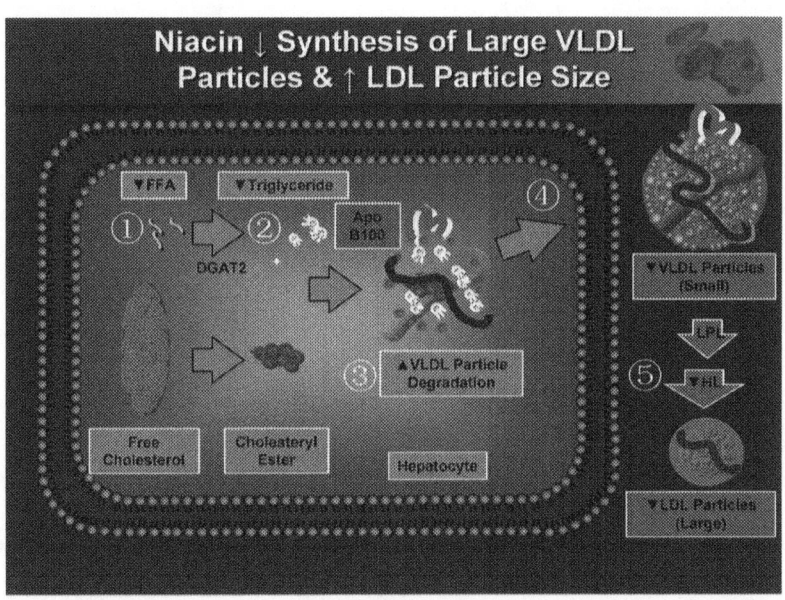

Image 36: Niacin ↓Synthesis of VLDL Particles
& Leads to Large LDL Particles

Niacin was the first agent ever used for lipoprotein disorders as well as the first lipid drug ever studied in terms of CV risk reduction, showing up to 25–30% prevention of otherwise preventable future CV events in a study of hundreds of patients. The only form of Niacin that can be recommended for use is prescription Niaspan (also found in combination with lovastatin in Advicor). All other forms of Niacin found on the market are dietary supplements without any FDA oversight whatsoever regarding safety, efficacy, quality, content or lot variability. Over-the-counter (OTC) Niacin products (where the FDA would be involved with oversight) DO NOT EXIST in the North American marketplace. Multiple medical authorities have warned against the use of dietary supplement Niacin, basically calling it weak, unsafe junk that "must not be used" (see Image 38 below). The forms of dietary supplement Niacin include: 1) nicotin-amide (completely ineffective); 2) immediate-release (poor quality); and 3) sustained release (less effective and associated with liver inflammation). For your information, prescription Niaspan is classified as an 'extended release' form of Niacin and is safe, effective and of top quality.

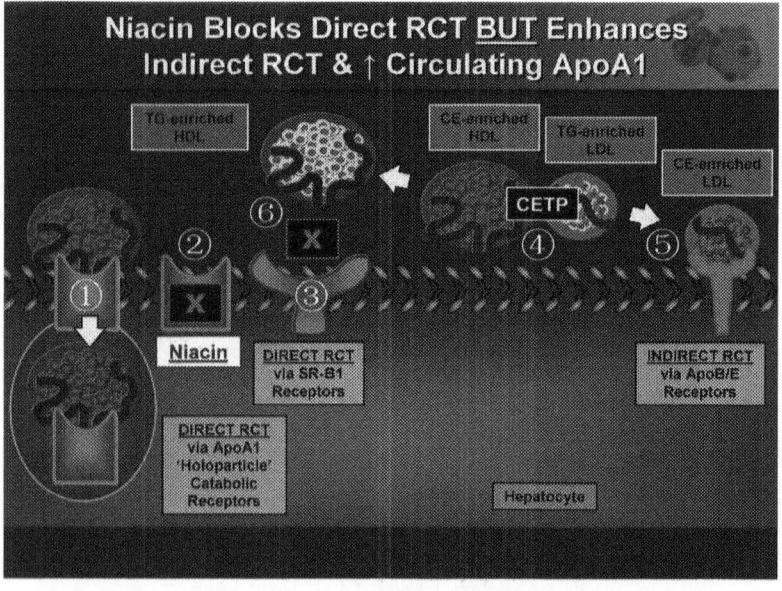

Image 37: Niacin Blocks Direct RCT BUT Enhances
Indirect RCT & ↑Circulating ApoA1

One other important benefit of Niacin therapy is its potent induction of vasodilatation (the opening of blood vessels). Niacin is one of the most powerful stimulators of endothelial nitric oxide synthetase (eNOS), an enzyme on the inner lining of blood vessels that causes them to relax and dilate (see Image 39 below). Individuals with CHD, type II DM, MS/IR and/or other states of high CV risk typically have low bloodstream levels of nitric oxide (NO) and are vasoconstricted as a result. The individual in this vasoconstricted state (which is harmful to the organs and tissues of the body) usually feels 'normal' since they are acclimated to the pathology. As Niacin quickly reverses this state, many patients who begin Niacin therapy initially experience 'flushing' complaints. These symptoms <u>ARE NOT</u> side effects, allergies or anything <u>BAD</u>. They are an expression of the patient changing from a pathologic vasoconstricted state to a physiologic vasodilated state. The page following the end of this chapter contains a copy of the instruction sheet that I give to my patients when I start them on Niaspan or Advicor therapy.

Fibrates are another drug class commonly prescribed for lipoprotein disorders. The safest and most effective Fibrate is probably Tricor. Like Statins and Niacin, Fibrates have multiple mechanisms of action. First and foremost, Fibrates decrease the production and enhance the clearance of VLDL particles (see Image 40 below). 1) Fibrates decrease intra-hepatic FFA levels available for TG synthesis. 2) Fibrates block the production of TG. 3) Fibrates thus lead to a decrease in the production of VLDL particles. 4) VLDL particle secretion slows with the particles being smaller with less TG in their core. 5) Fibrates also increase lipoprotein lipase (LPL) levels and decrease Apo-CIII levels, converting the small, TG-poor VLDL particles into large, CE-rich LDL particles rather quickly. Fibrates should not be taken by individuals with liver problems and should be used with caution by individuals with kidney problems.

Fibrates directly act upon PPARα to decrease VLDL particle production and enhance VLDL particle clearance (see Image 41 below). 1) Fibrates stimulate PPARα within the nucleus of many cells, including hepatocytes. 2) This leads to a decrease in the expression of ApoC-III which would otherwise block ApoE recognition by hepatic LRP receptors. In this manner, Fibrates directly enhance VLDL particle removal from the bloodstream. 3) PPARα stimulation also increases the genetic expression of LPL which can thereby remove TG from VLDL particles (in the absence of ApoC-III which would otherwise block ApoC-II interaction with LPL). 4) TG is removed from VLDL particles and converted into FFA. 5) The FFA is taken up by muscle cells and metabolized to generate cellular energy. 6) The FFA is also taken up by adipocytes and converted into TG for storage. 7) The FFA also enters hepatocytes. 8) There FFA is metabolized in such a manner as to decrease TG synthesis. 9) Decreased TG levels in the hepatocyte lead to reduced VLDL particle production and secretion. 10) Note that Niacin blocks the release of FFA from adipocytes into the circulation as mentioned above.

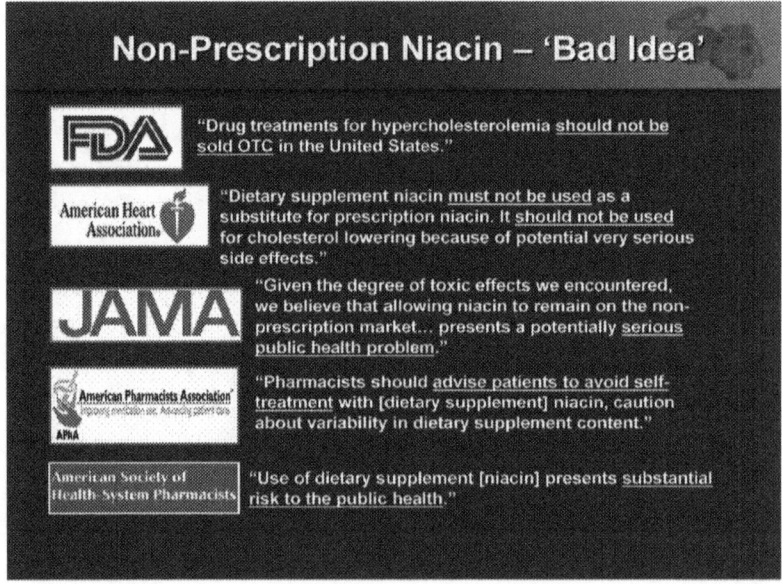

Image 38: Non-Prescription Niacin—'Bad Idea'

Fibrates also have potent effects upon HDL particle dynamics (see Image 42 below). Fibrates directly stimulate PPARα within the nucleus of the hepatocyte. 1) This induces the expression of the ApoA1 gene (1) as well as the ApoA2 gene (2). Both ApoA1 (3) and ApoA2 (4) are thus manufactured. 5) Nascent HDL particles containing ApoA1 are secreted into the bloodstream. 6) ApoA2 assists in the maturation of HDL particles after being transferred onto them by various β-lipoproteins. 7) Circulating HDL particles tend to be small on Fibrate therapy since, as soon as they become large and CE-enriched, they are recognized by hepatic SR-B1 receptors (also up-regulated by Fibrate therapy) and rapidly de-lipidated.

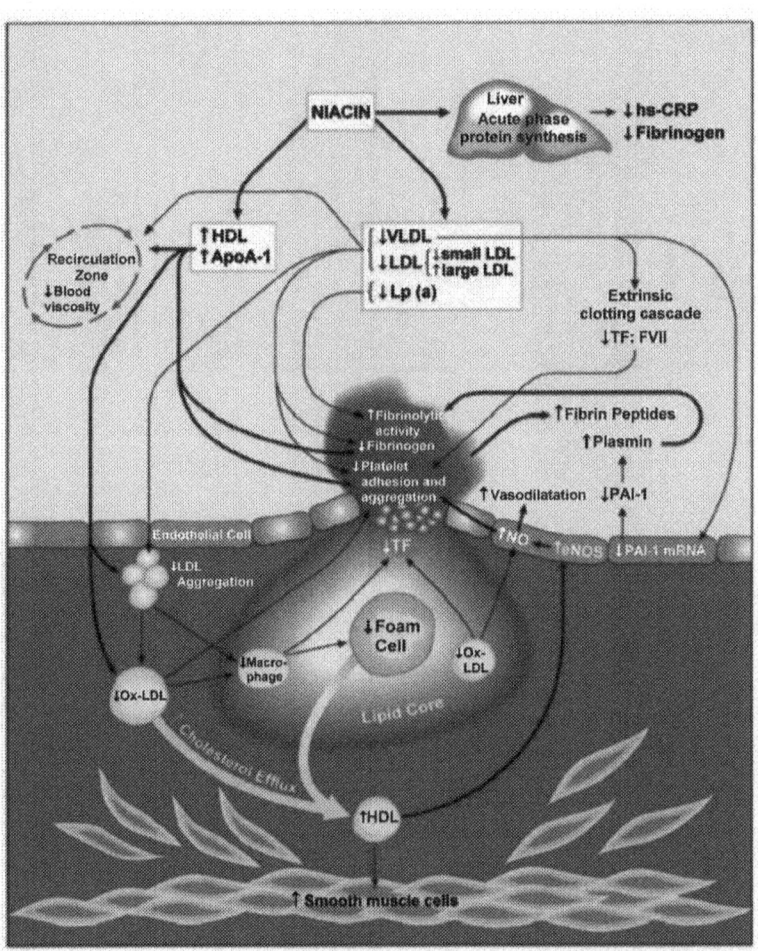

Image 39: Physiologic Benefits of Niacin

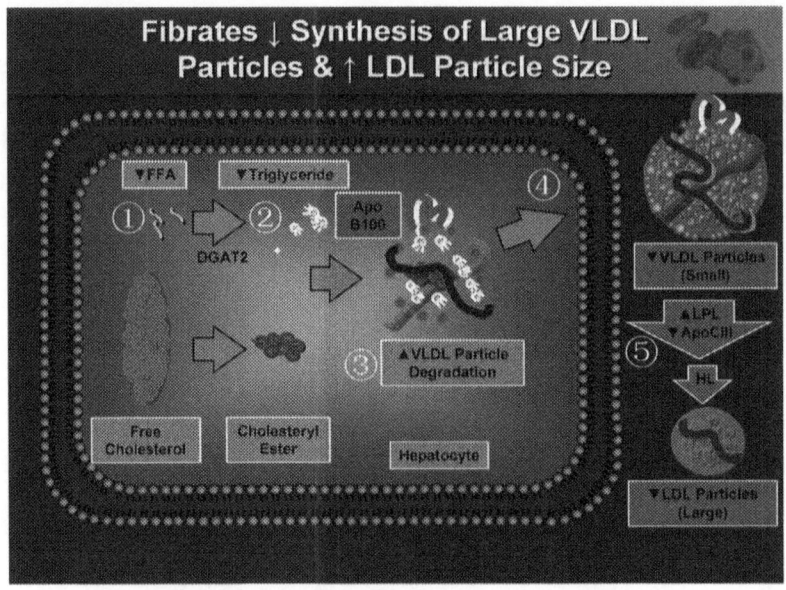

Image 40: Fibrates ↓Synthesis of VLDL
Particles & ↑LDL Particle Size

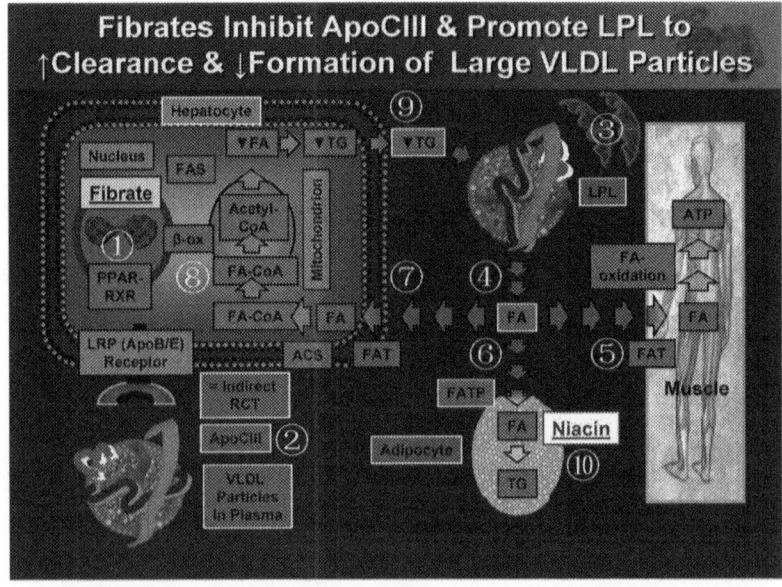

Image 41: Fibrates Inhibit ApoC-III & Promote LPL to
↓Formation & ↑Clearance of Large VLDL Particles

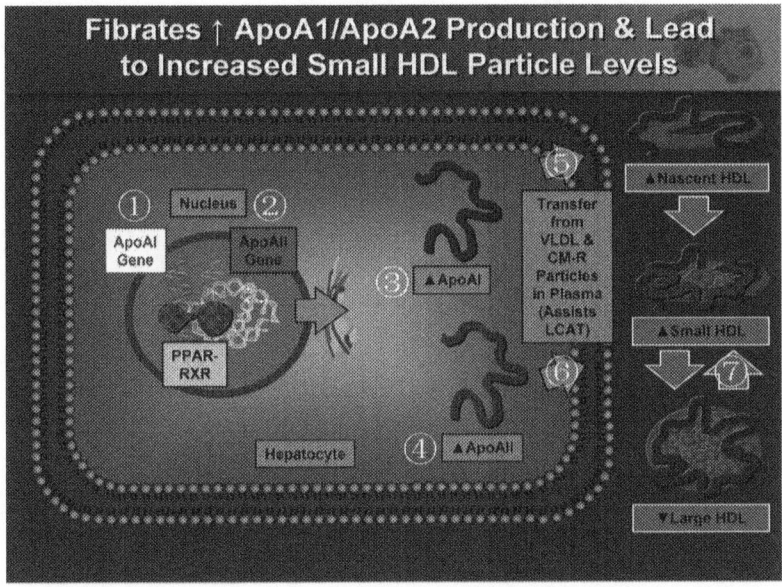

Image 42: Fibrates ↑ApoA1/ApoA2 Production & Lead
to Increased Small HDL Particle Levels

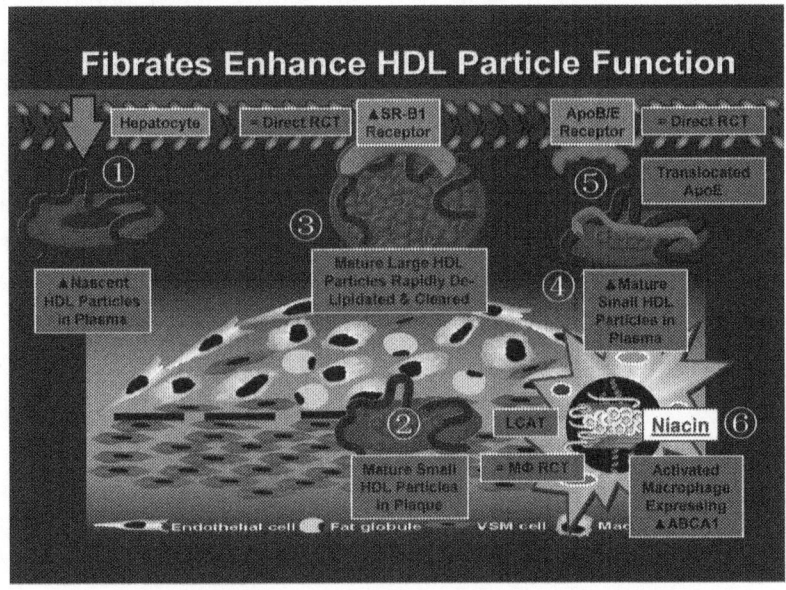

Image 43: Fibrates Enhance HDL Particle Function

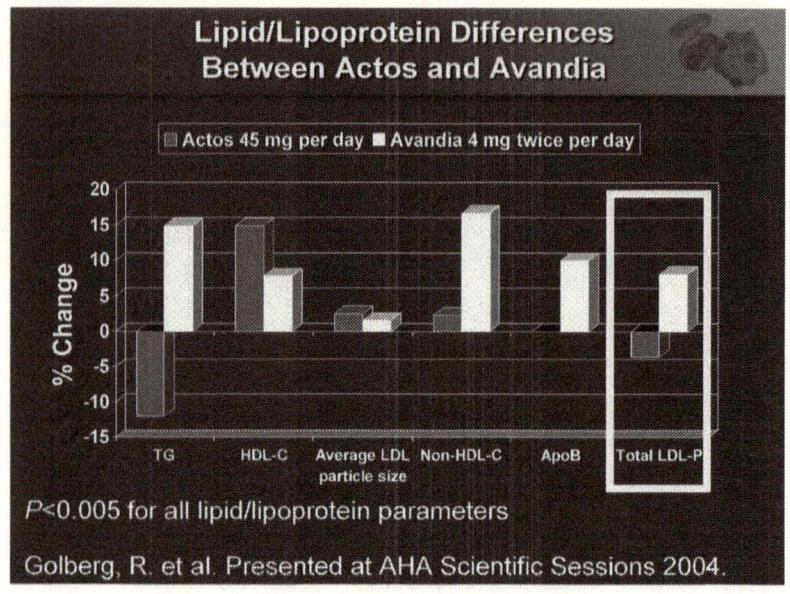

Image 44: Lipid/Lipoprotein Differences
Between Actos and Avandia

Fibrates enhance HDL particle function (see Image 43 above). 1) Fibrates increase nascent HDL particle release from hepatocytes. 2) These particles penetrate into atherosclerotic plaques where ATP Binding Cassette A1 (ABCA1—also enhanced with Fibrate therapy) transfers FC from activated macrophages into them. LCAT (lecithin cholesterol acyl-transferase) converts the FC into CE (with the help of ApoA2) and the nascent HDL particles become mature. 3) Fibrates up-regulate SR-B1 receptors which recognize and de-lipidate mature large HDL particles in the process of direct RCT. 4) Mature small HDL particles are not rec-ognized by SR-B1. 5) Mature small HDL particles can be removed from circulation by ApoB/E receptors if they contain translocated ApoE. 6) Note that Niacin can also induce the production and function of ABCA1 within activated macrophages in atherosclerotic plaques.

Fibrates have prevented 20–30% of otherwise preventable CV events in clinical outcome studies involving thousands of patients. Glitazones (Actos, Avandia) function similar to Fibrates in terms of PPARα stimulation. Actos seems to be the preferable Glitazone since it is equally safe and effective in terms of blood sugar control but far superior in terms of lipid/lipoprotein effects (see Image 44 above). Note that Actos lowers total LDL-P while Avandia actually increases it. Think of Statins as Batman: we know that Batman always wins. But wouldn't you rather have Batman and Robin (Actos which helps by further lowering total LDL-P) than Batman and the Joker (Avandia which fights by increasing total LDL-P)?

Prescription fish oils function by inhibiting TG synthesis (1) as well as blocking the formation (2) and secretion (3) of VLDL particles (both large as well as small—see Image 45 below). This will decrease circulating levels of VLDL particles as well as IDL/LDL particles (to a lesser extent). Prescription Omacor should now be the form used rather than any dietary supplement having no FDA oversight whatsoever regarding safety, efficacy, quality (especially in terms of whether oxidation of DHA/EPA has occurred—which is what causes fish to smell 'fishy'), content (especially in terms of possible mercury contamination—highest in swordfish and lowest in krill) or lot variability.

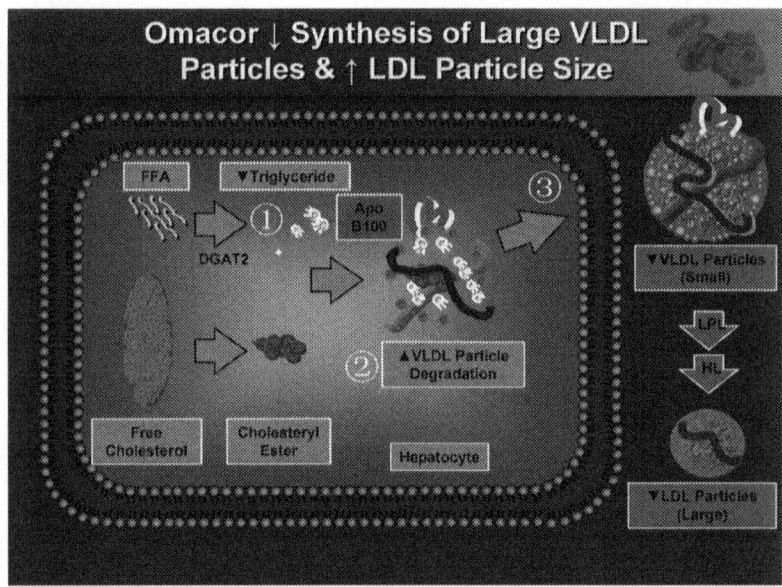

Image 45: Omacor ↓Synthesis of VLDL
Particles & ↑LDL Particle Size

Please remember that lipid-modifying medications (regardless of which ones) only work in the long run if they are added to an appropriate lifestyle. Such medications aren't like Jack's magic beans—if you turn yourself into the giant, they don't work so well. Medications can work well as 'supplements' to common sense; they usually work poorly as 'substitutes.' Imagine a stock pot full of water, boiling over. Taking any lipid medication is like putting a lid on the pot. Losing weight, eating right and exercising is like turning down the heat. You turn down the heat as much as you can and, if the pot is still boiling over, <u>THEN</u> you put on the lid. If you never turn down the heat, heavier and heavier lids (more and more lipid-modifying medications) will be required over time—only to delay the pot from inevitably boiling over and making a big mess.

I have always recognized that medications for HTN, type II DM and/ or dyslipoproteinemia are many times not even required if people 'do what they need to do'—become slender, live an active daily lifestyle, eat proper amount of 'healthy' food and limit their intake of 'junk' food. Even if medications do prove necessary, as long as the individual follows this heart-healthy, common sense lifestyle, usually only low doses of limited numbers of medications will be required. However, if the individual is overweight, overstressed, sedentary, consumes excessive calories and/ or limited amounts of micronutrients, medications definitely will prove necessary with more and more required as time passes, typically following the law of diminishing return.

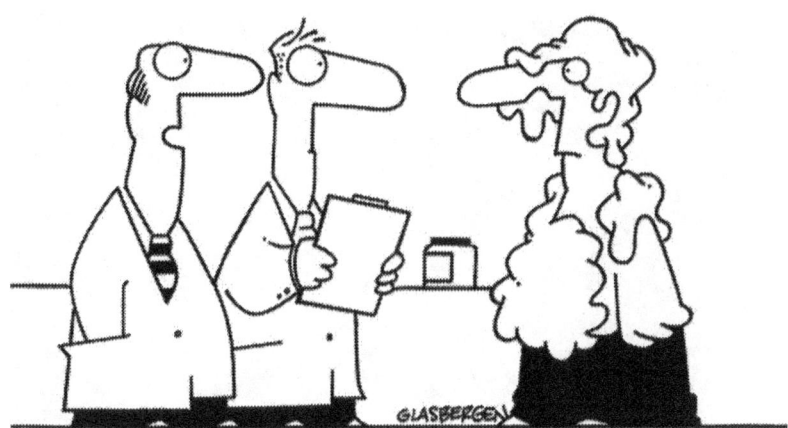

"With this new drug, cholesterol forms outside of the body, where it can't clog the arteries!"

Part II. Putting It All Together

We will now put together all the concepts detailed in this book and use them in the analysis of an actual patient case (see Image 46 below). Our patient is a 57 year-old postmenopausal woman with a significant family history of premature CHD as well as a significant personal medical history of HTN. Obviously she has a relatively high future risk of experiencing CV-related events and/or of developing type II DM. She has no CV complaints but we know that 75% of people who experience their first heart attack never have previous chest discomfort symptoms. She currently takes a blood pressure medication called Cardizem LA as well as low-dose aspirin and some vitamins. She has never smoked nor abused alcohol but does not exercise, is otherwise fairly sedentary (walking around 2000–3000 steps per day) and eats 'junk' just like many of the rest of us. Her resting blood pressure and pulse are fairly well controlled. She weighs 175# and is 5'5" tall with a 38" waist. Her baseline labs appear normal.

Image 46: Sample Patient Case #4—Baseline

We order advanced lipid testing (for sake of discussion we will show SGGE, VAP as well as NMR results). Baseline SGGE lipid testing (see Image 47 below) shows low-risk TC, HDL-C, TG, Lp(a), homocysteine, ApoE genotype and fibrinogen with intermediate-risk LDL-C, high-sensitivity CRP and insulin as well as high-risk LDL IIIa+b and IVb (small LDL particles), HDL 2b (large HDL particles), ApoB and Lp-PLA$_2$. Baseline VAP lipid testing (see Image 48 below) shows normal TC, total direct LDL-C, total direct HDL-C, direct TG, total direct non-HDL-C and 'real' LDL-C but shows elevated total direct VLDL-C, Lp(a)-C, IDL-C and pattern B real LDL (indicating increased amounts of small LDL particles) and remnant lipoproteins. Baseline NMR lipoprotein testing (see Image 49 below) shows near-optimal risk LDL-C and otherwise normal TC, HDL-C and TG but shows very high-risk total LDL-P of 2310 nmol/L with high-risk small LDL-P of 1730 nmol/L as well as all three abnormal lipoprotein characteristics (elevated small LDL-P, elevated large VLDL-P and low large HDL-P) suggestive of MS/IR as well as serving as the foundation for the possible later development of type II DM (see Image 16). Thus all three advanced lipid tests demonstrate this patient to have elevated risk of future CV events (due mainly to increased small LDL particles) despite traditional lipid testing appearing 'normal.'

		Normal	Inter-mediate	At Risk	Last Visit	Alert Value	ATP III Goal	Reference Range
NCEP ATP III Lipid Tests	Total Cholesterol (mg/dL)	184				>/= 200 mg/dL	< 200	129-321
	LDL-C (mg/dL)		109			>/= 130 mg/dL	< 100	58-148
	HDL-C (mg/dL)	46				< 40 mg/dL	> 40	32-60
	Triglycerides (mg/dL)	145				> 150 mg/dL	< 150	60-263
		Normal	Inter-mediate	At Risk	Last Visit	Alert Value	SHL Goal	Reference Range
Advanced Cardiovascular Risk Markers	IIIa+b (%)			74.1		>=20	<=15	13.6-43.0
	LDL IVb (%)			16.0		>=10	<=5	1.7-9.8
	HDL 2b (%)			3.5		<10	>20	7-30
	ApoB (mg/dL)			135		>120	<60	60-340
	Extended Range Lp(a) (mg/dL)	20.4				>=30	<30	0-30
	Homocysteine (mmol/L)	8.0				>=14	<10	5.0-12.0
	ApoE genotype	3/3				3/4, 4/4	3/3	
	C-Reactive Protein (mg/dL)		2.8			>3.0	<1.0	0.0-1.69
	Lp-PLA2 (mg/dL)			212		>=200	<200	
	Fibrinogen (mg/dL)	265				>=350	<350	180-350
	Insulin (nU/mL)		11.9			>=12	<10	6-27

Image 47: Sample Patient Case #4—Baseline SGGE

Baseline CIMT testing demonstrates this woman to have significant soft plaque at both common carotid artery (CCA) bifurcations (see Image 50 below). Her average CCA mean CIMT is 0.921 mm which is compatible with that of an average woman greater than 80 years of age. Thus this woman already has evidence of rather significant atherosclerosis.

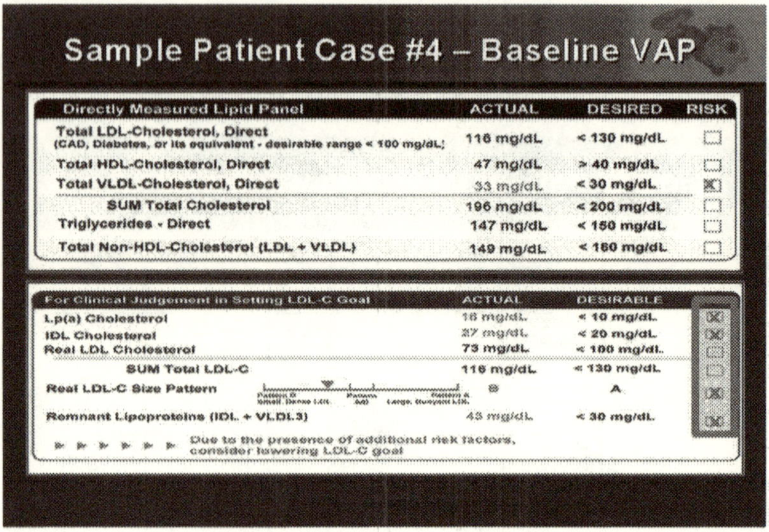

Image 48: Sample Patient Case #4—Baseline VAP

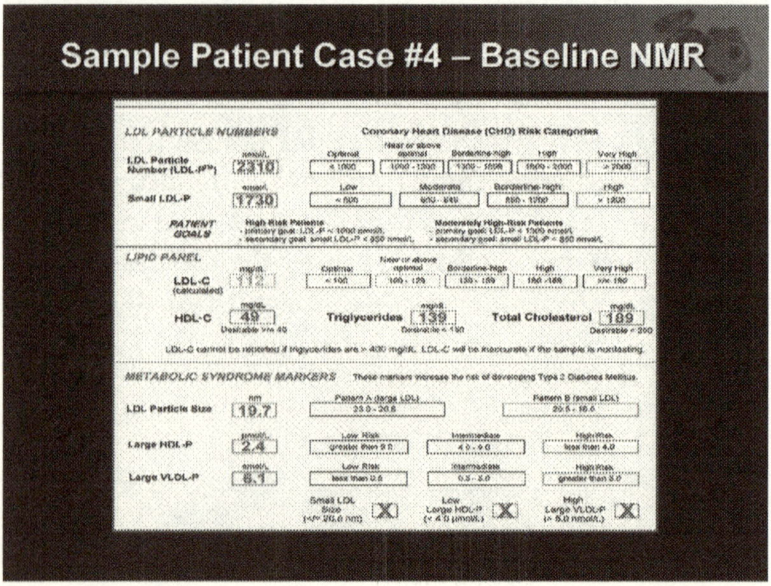

Image 49: Sample Patient Case #4—Baseline NMR

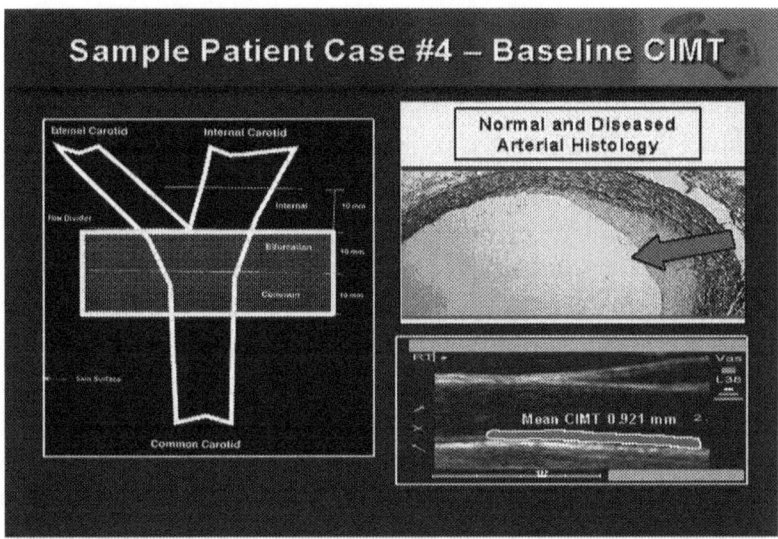

Image 50: Sample Patient Case #4—Baseline CIMT

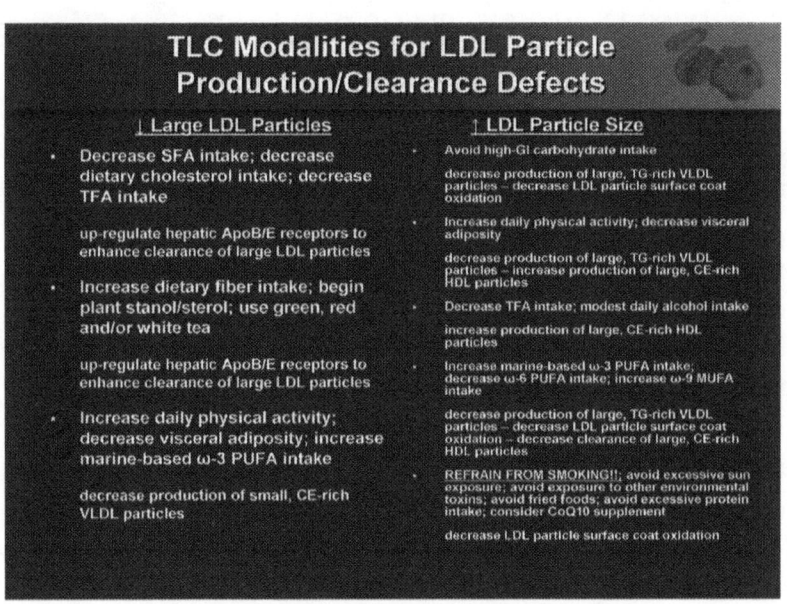

Image 51: TLC Modalities for LDL Particle
Production/Clearance Defects

When total LDL-P is higher than goal (which in this woman would be < 1000–1300 nmol/L), it is imperative to determine what specific type of lipoprotein abnormality is at fault. Obviously her total LDL-P is elevated because of the small LDL particles much more so than the large LDL particles.

We therefore recommend three to six months of therapeutic lifestyle changes (TLC) to get her total LDL-P to goal (see Image 51 above). We first suggest: 1) decreasing intake of TFA, SFA and dietary cholesterol and beginning a fiber supplement, green tea as well as Benecol—to up-regulate hepatic ApoB/E receptors and remove excess large LDL particles from the bloodstream; and 2) decreasing intake of high-GI carbohydrates (other than right around the time of exercise), losing weight and increasing daily physical activity as well as marine-based ω-3 PUFA intake—to decrease small VLDL particle production and thus the levels of large LDL particles.

But our patient's problem is not elevated levels of large LDL particles—it is elevated levels of small LDL particles. So we also recommend: 1) MODEST daily alcohol intake (no more than 1 oz) to increase large HDL particles; 2) increasing ω-9 MUFA intake and decreasing ω-6 PUFA intake to decrease large VLDL particles, increase large HDL particles and decrease LDL particle surface coat oxidation; as well as 3) avoiding fried foods, limiting protein/sodium/caffeine intake, reducing personal stress level (easier said than done) and considering a CoQ10 supplement to decrease LDL particle surface coat oxidation. All these changes will help increase LDL particle size. By the way, the best way to limit lipoprotein particle surface coat oxidation is to REFRAIN FROM SMOKING!

We inform our patient that her IBW is 130# (see Table 3) and suggest that her total basal caloric consumption based on her daily activity level should be around 1400–1600 calories per day (see Table 4). Our patient follows all our advice, starts the 'HAPI Heart Diet' and loses 26# over six months (see Image 52 below). She now walks at least 10,000 steps per day. Her resting blood pressure and pulse have decreased. She tells us that she feels "way better and much healthier than in a long, long time."

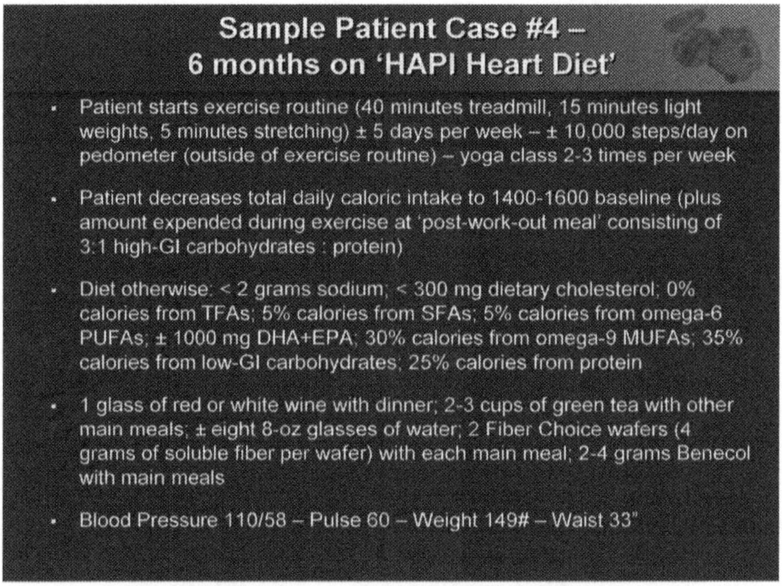

Image 52: Sample Patient Case #4—6 months
on 'HAPI Heart Diet'

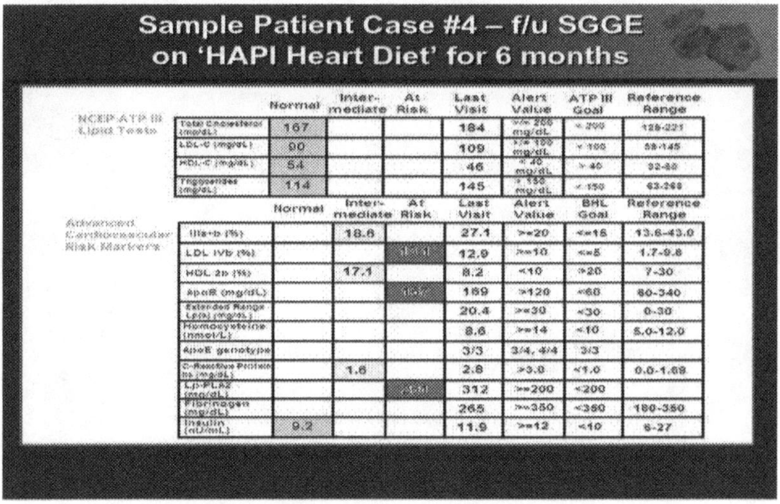

Image 53: Sample Patient Case #4—f/u SGGE
on 'HAPI Heart Diet' for 6 months

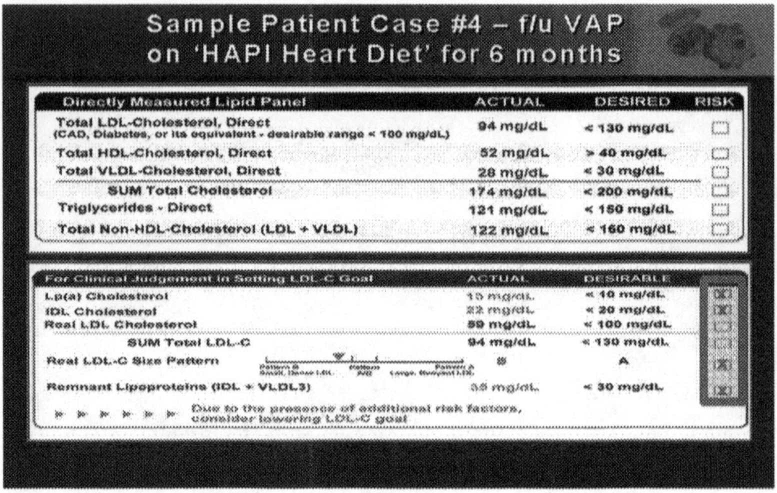

Image 54: Sample Patient Case #4—f/u VAP
on 'HAPI Heart Diet' for 6 months

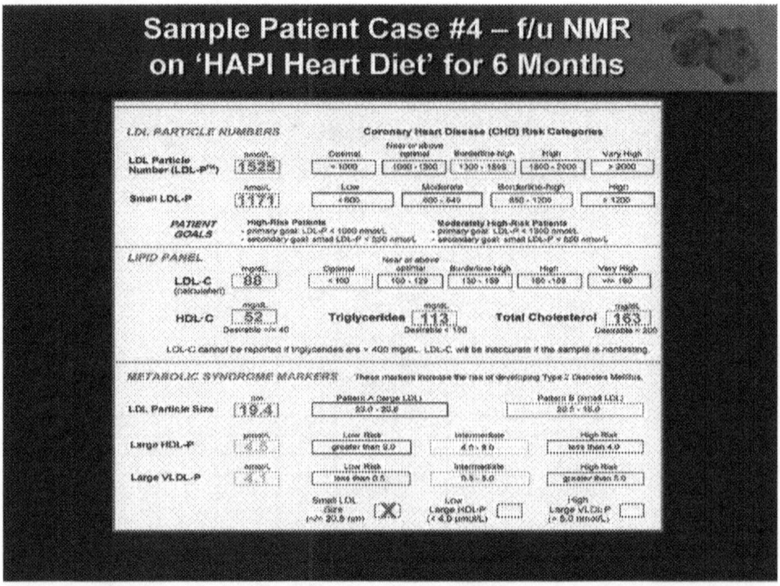

Image 55: Sample Patient Case #4—f/u NMR
on 'HAPI Heart Diet' for 6 months

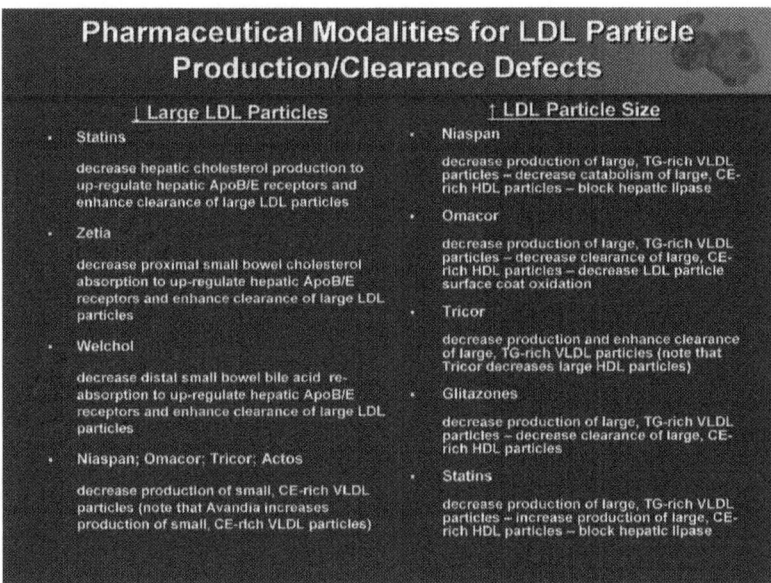

Image 56: Pharmaceutical Modalities for LDL Particle
Production/Clearance Defects

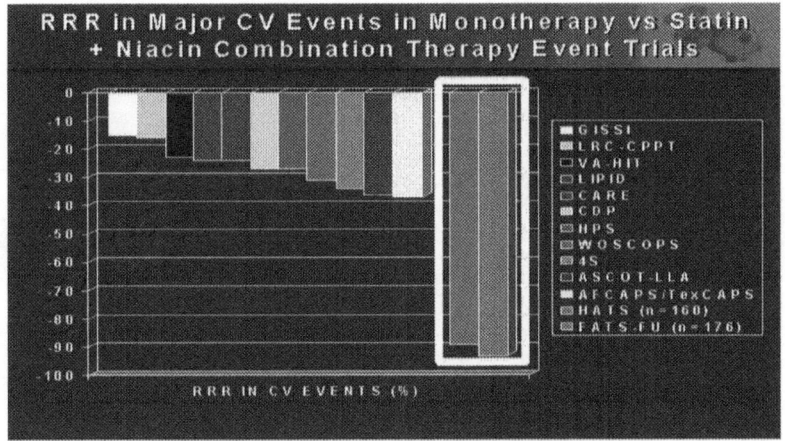

Image 57: RRR in Major CV Events in Monotherapy vs
Statin + Niacin Combination Therapy Trials

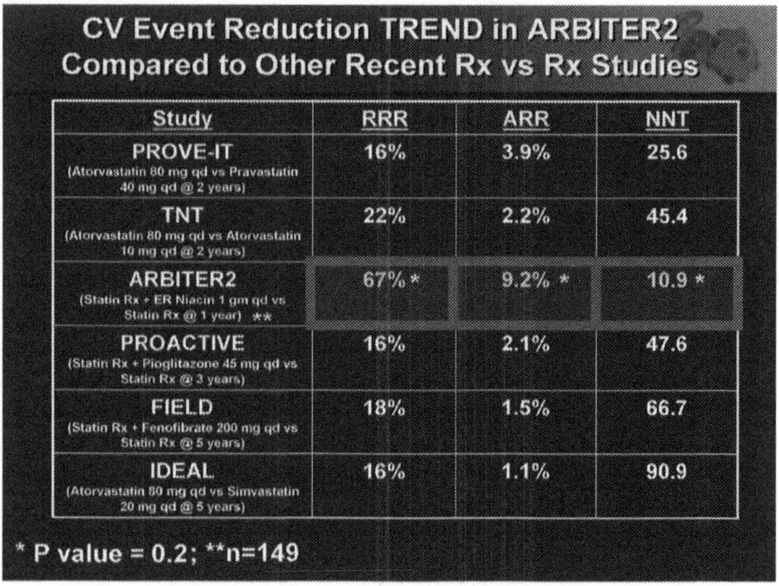

CV Event Reduction TREND in ARBITER2 Compared to Other Recent Rx vs Rx Studies

Study	RRR	ARR	NNT
PROVE-IT (Atorvastatin 80 mg qd vs Pravastatin 40 mg qd @ 2 years)	16%	3.9%	25.6
TNT (Atorvastatin 80 mg qd vs Atorvastatin 10 mg qd @ 2 years)	22%	2.2%	45.4
ARBITER2 (Statin Rx + ER Niacin 1 gm qd vs Statin Rx @ 1 year) **	67% *	9.2% *	10.9 *
PROACTIVE (Statin Rx + Pioglitazone 45 mg qd vs Statin Rx @ 3 years)	16%	2.1%	47.6
FIELD (Statin Rx + Fenofibrate 200 mg qd vs Statin Rx @ 5 years)	18%	1.5%	66.7
IDEAL (Atorvastatin 80 mg qd vs Simvastatin 20 mg qd @ 5 years)	16%	1.1%	90.9

* P value = 0.2; **n=149

Image 58: CV Event Reduction TREND in ARBITER2 Compared to Other Recent Rx vs Rx Studies

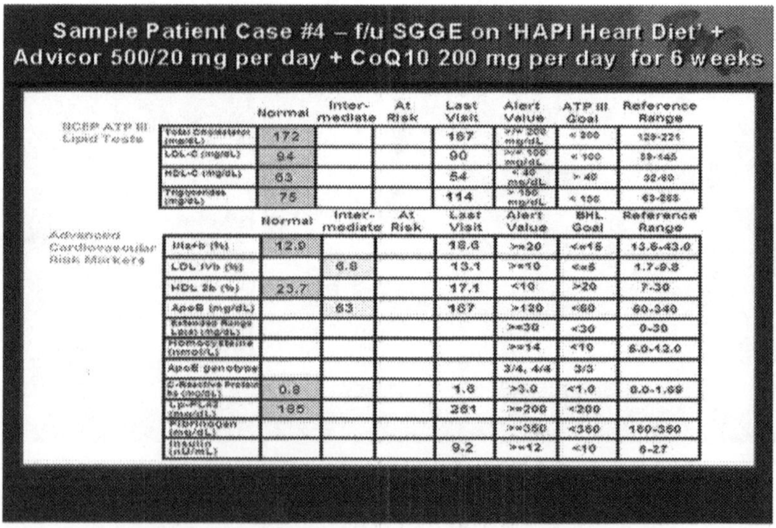

Sample Patient Case #4 – f/u SGGE on 'HAPI Heart Diet' + Advicor 500/20 mg per day + CoQ10 200 mg per day for 6 weeks

NCEP ATP III Lipid Tests

	Normal	Inter-mediate	At Risk	Last Visit	Alert Value	ATP III Goal	Reference Range
Total Cholesterol (mg/dL)	172			167	>= 200 mg/dL	< 200	129-221
LDL-C (mg/dL)	94			90	>= 100 mg/dL	< 100	59-145
HDL-C (mg/dL)	63			54	< 40 mg/dL	> 40	32-60
Triglycerides (mg/dL)	75			114	> 150 mg/dL	< 150	63-283

Advanced Cardiovascular Risk Markers

	Normal	Inter-mediate	At Risk	Last Visit	Alert Value	BHL Goal	Reference Range
IIIa+b (%)	12.9			18.6	>=20	<=15	13.6-43.0
LDL IVb (%)		6.8		13.1	>=10	<=5	1.7-9.8
HDL 2b (%)	23.7			17.1	<10	>20	7-30
ApoB (mg/dL)		63		167	>120	<80	60-340
Extended Range Lp(a) (mg/dL)					>=30	<30	0-30
Homocysteine (umol/L)					>=14	<10	5.0-12.0
ApoE genotype					3/4, 4/4	3/3	
C-Reactive Protein hs (mg/dL)	0.8			1.6	>3.0	<1.0	0.0-1.69
Lp-PLA2 (ng/mL)	185			261	>=200	<200	
Fibrinogen (mg/dL)					>=350	<350	180-350
Insulin (uU/mL)				9.2	>=12	<10	6-27

Image 59: Sample Patient Case #4—f/u SGGE on 'HAPI Heart Diet' + Advicor 500/20 mg per day + CoQ10 200 mg per day for 6 weeks

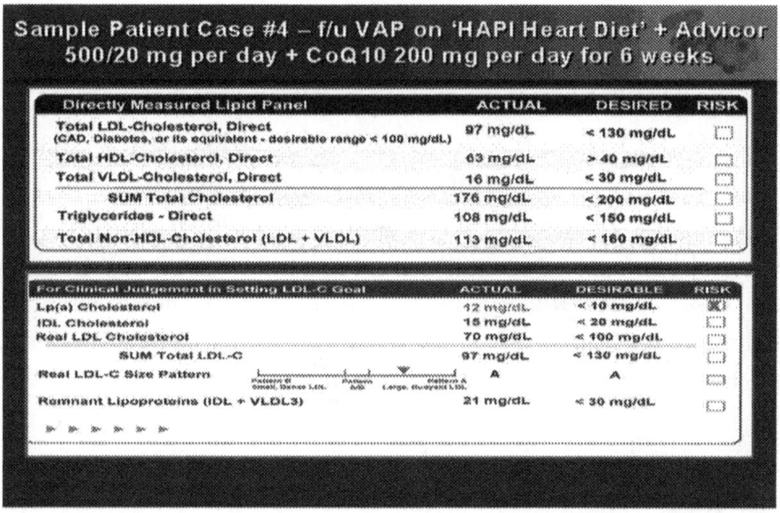

Image 60: Sample Patient Case #4—f/u VAP on 'HAPI Heart Diet' + Advicor 500/20 mg per day + CoQ10 200 mg per day for 6 weeks

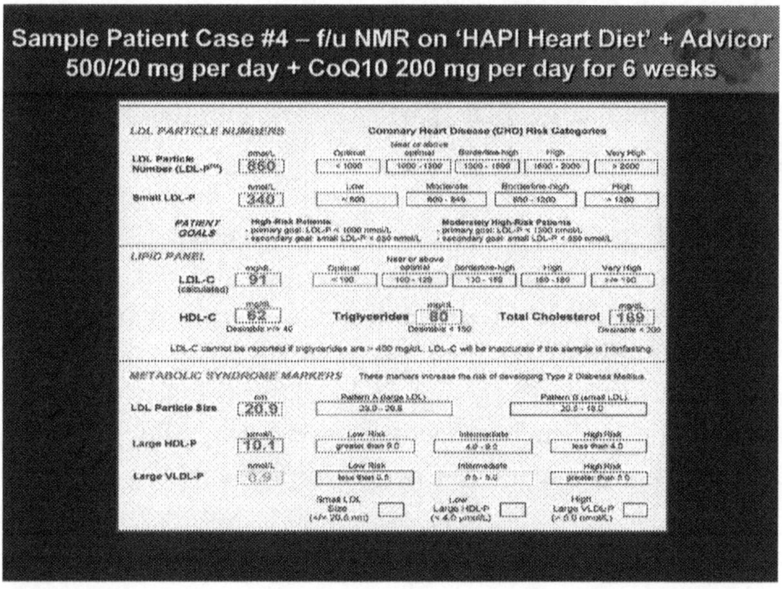

Image 61: Sample Patient Case #4—f/u NMR on 'HAPI Heart Diet' + Advicor 500/20 mg per day + CoQ10 200 mg per day for 6 weeks

We repeat advanced lipid testing to determine what has changed from this perspective. SGGE, VAP and NMR testing all demonstrate interval improvement in lipoprotein subclass parameters (see Images 53, 54, 55 above). Her total LDL-P has dropped to 1525 nmol with a small LDL-P of 1171 nmol/L. This means her CHD risk is better than when we first saw her but she still has relatively high likelihood of future CV-related events. Her LDL-C is once again underestimating the real problem (by almost 100%) and 'lying' to us. We are pleased that she now has just one of the three lipoprotein manifestations of pre-diabetes (the iceberg seems to be melting along with her waistline).

Since she is not yet at her total LDL-P goal and TLC did not work to optimize her CV risk by six months (although all values have definitely improved when compared to her baseline), we realize this probably is the time to add appropriate pharmaceutical therapy.

The most potent lipid-modifying drugs for up-regulating ApoB/E receptors to clear large LDL particles from the bloodstream are Statins, Zetia and BAS/Welchol (in that order—see Image 56 above). The most potent agents to decrease the formation of small VLDL particles (which are converted into large LDL particles) are Fibrates/Tricor, Niaspan, Omacor, Actos, Statins and Zetia.

We obviously must increase our patient's average LDL particle size. The most powerful drugs in decreasing large VLDL particles are Tricor, Omacor, Niaspan, Actos, Statins and Zetia. The most potent pharmaceuticals in increasing large HDL particles are Niaspan, Glitazones and Statins. The most powerful drugs in blocking the function of HL are Niaspan and Statins. The best agents in preventing LDL particle surface coat oxidation are Omacor and CoQ10 supplements.

Thus Statins are the best drugs to remove large LDL particles whereas Niaspan seems a great choice to increase average LDL particle size. Three small clinical outcome trials involving Statin + Niacin combination therapy (HATS, FATS-FU and ARBITER2—see Images 57 and 58 above) showed rather impressive results. We therefore recommend the addition of Advicor as well as a high-quality CoQ10 supplement to the 'HAPI Heart Diet.' Other equally appropriate pharmacologic choices could obviously have been made (such as Statin + Tricor (based on the FIELD trial results and the very large number of patients in Fibrate trials [second only to Statin trials]); Statin + Omacor (based on the GISSI trial results); Zetia + Fibrate; Zetia + Niaspan; or Zetia + Omacor).

A Word on the Importance of Ubiquinone

The most powerful antioxidant in the human body is ubiquinone (Coenzyme Q10 or CoQ10) which scavenges extra electrons from oxidative substances such as free radicals (created from smoking, excessive sun exposure, environmental toxins, eating fried foods, consuming excessive refined carbohydrates, protein, caffeine and/or sodium) and shuttles those electrons to the cell's internal mitochondria to assist in energy production. Supplementation with CoQ10 at 100 mg per day was studied in patients with advanced (class 3 and class 4) congestive heart failure (Folkers, Karl et. al. <u>Biomedical and Clinical Aspects of Coenzyme Q10</u>. Vol. 5. 1986) and demonstrated a 50% absolute reduction in all-cause mortality at one year. Compare this to the SOLVD study (*NEJM*. 1991:325;293–302) using the ACE-inhibitor enalapril on patients with Class 2 and Class 3 congestive heart failure where enalapril-treated patients had a 3.25% absolute risk reduction in death at one year. ACE-inhibitors are now considered a mainstay of medical treatment for congestive heart failure whereas the potential benefit of CoQ10 supplementation has basically been ignored and even ridiculed by the medical establishment.

Note that the aging process seems to lower ubiquinone levels and that Statin medications block the production of CoQ10 (decreasing its content within β-lipoproteins by at least 50%). A study (Bargossis, AM et al. *Molec. Aspects Med.* 1994:15;187–193) involving patients taking Zocor (a Statin) at a dose of 20 mg per day showed their plasma CoQ10 levels drop 27.7% after 90 days. When similar patients were also begun on 100 mg of CoQ10 per day, their plasma CoQ10 levels actually increased 23.3%. Another study (Palomaki, A et al. *Journ. of Lipid Research.* 1998:39;1430–1437) showed that patients taking Mevacor (another Statin) at 60 mg per day along with CoQ10 at 180 mg per day had a 400% increase in LDL particle CoQ10 levels compared to patients taking Mevacor alone.

As CoQ10 helps prevent oxidative injury to lipoprotein surface coats, it also helps prevent the formation of small LDL particles and small HDL particles. In my own practice, I recommend that anyone on Statin-based medical therapy also consider taking a good-quality CoQ10 supplement (such as Q-Gel at 100–300 mg per day). Note that the absorption of CoQ10 from the gut is dependent upon taking it with a fatty meal.

There are those clinicians who are very skeptical regarding the results of the Statin + Niacin CV event trials—arguing that they were of small sample size (only around 150 to 175 individuals in each) and larger trials would be necessary in order to consider Statin + Niacin a new 'core' therapy for dyslipoproteinemia. However, what's the upside (perhaps up to 90–95% prevention of otherwise preventable CV events)? What's the downside ('flushing' which actually represents another real clinical benefit—the opening of otherwise closed blood vessels)? What do you think? If you get 20 doctors in one room, you'll have 40+ opinions—that's for sure. Obviously, we'll all have to wait until the large scale combination therapy trials are published (Statin + CETP inhibitor versus

Statin; Statin + Tricor versus Statin; and Statin + Niaspan versus Statin) to really know the 'truth.'

After six weeks of medical therapy on top of the 'HAPI Heart Diet,' our patient returns and we repeat advanced lipid testing (see Images 59, 60, 61 above). Things now look <u>GREAT</u> with total LDL-P of 860 nmol/L and small LDL-P of 340 nmol/L. Her risk for future CV events as well as the development of type II DM is now quite low and thus optimal. We are happy since our patient now has a much healthier heart. Note the LDL-C went up 3–4 mg/dL when the actual total LDL-P dropped by almost 100%. How worthless LDL-C testing was in this individual!

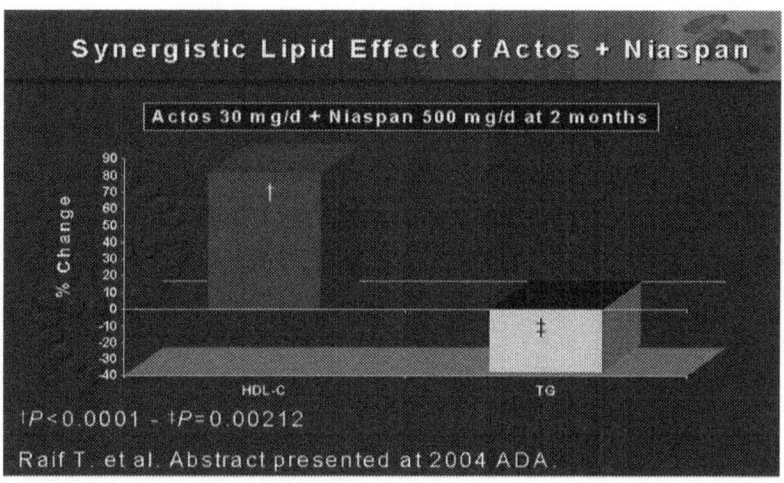

Image 62: Synergistic Lipid Effects of Actos + Niaspan

By the way, if the total LDL-P on Advicor would have remained above goal due to increased large LDL-P, our options would have included: 1) increasing lovastatin dose; 2) changing lovastatin to a more powerful Statin; 3) adding Zetia [this would be suggested by a significant increase in the serum campesterol to lathosterol ratio—which can be ordered through Mayo Clinic]; and/or 4) adding Welchol. On the contrary, if the total LDL-P would have remained above goal due to increased small LDL-P, our options would have been: 1) giving it some more time

(Niaspan's effect upon HDL-C and LDL particle size improves over time); 2) increasing Niaspan dose; 3) adding Omacor; 4) adding Tricor; and/or 5) adding Actos. The most powerful of these approaches might be adding Actos to the Advicor. A fairly recent trial in type 2 diabetics with IR showed the combination of Actos at 30 mg per day with Niaspan at 500 mg per day increased HDL-C by 81.5% and decreased TG by 37% at two months (thus increasing LDL particle size—see Image 62 above). Picture the family Thanksgiving feast with the Statin and Niaspan sitting at the 'grown-ups' table and Actos, Omacor, Tricor, Welchol and Zetia sitting at the 'kids' table. Sometimes there's room at the adult table for one (or more) of the kids: Welchol and/or Zetia might sit next to the Statin (if there's room) while Actos, Omacor and/or Tricor might sit next to Niaspan (if there's room).

Please realize there is one major drawback to advanced lipid testing (or for that matter to any form of lipid testing). TGs are carried both by endogenous particles (made by the liver—mainly VLDL particles, especially large VLDL particles) as well as by exogenous particles (made in the gut—chylomicron particles and CM-R particles). The reason we do an eight to 12 hour fast before checking lipoproteins (or lipids) is to rid the exogenous particles from the bloodstream to focus on what the liver is making. In the normal physiologic state, the exogenous particles have a half-life of about two to three hours, thus the typical eight to 12 hour fast will be sufficient to rid them from the bloodstream. But we're not talking about people with normal physiology, are we? We're talking about people with MS/IR where they have impairment of LPL due to elevated FFA levels and thus impairment of TG clearance from TG-containing lipoprotein particles, whether endogenous OR exogenous.

When we do the 'typical' eight to 12 hour fast and measure VLDL particles (especially the large ones) or TG, we might actually be measuring what that person ate (or drank) yesterday. Medications focus on what the liver makes while ONLY lifestyle changes will really effect what the gut is absorbing/producing. So, whenever you have a patient with very elevated 'fasting' VLDL particles or TG, I recommend a prolonged 24 to 36 hour fast (including <u>NO</u> alcohol), and then recheck the SGGE/VAP/NMR. You'll be amazed at what you see. I've <u>ROUTINELY</u> seen patients drop from TG levels over 10,000 mg/dL to levels more like 200–250 mg/dL. Since few people will actually tolerate a 24 to 36 hour water-only fast, I compromise by suggesting 12 hours of no caloric intake preceded by 12 to 24 hours of only very light, small meals and definitely no alcohol. When the VLDL particles or TG levels drop dramatically, I work with the patient to find out what particular dietary/lifestyle indiscretion is causing this.

We'll repeat the fast later (perhaps checking TG alone) except the patient will either drink the two glasses of red wine with a light dinner or have the big, juicy steak at dinner or have the big plateful of pasta at dinner or have the big bowl of ice cream just before going to bed. If the TG levels skyrocket, we've identified the problem and the patient just <u>CAN'T</u> do it anymore since their body just can't handle it. If the TG levels don't skyrocket, we'll keep checking until we find the culprit(s).

Once fasting total LDL-P and small LDL-P appear optimal for the individual patient, it's probably not a bad idea to 'double-check your work' with Lp-PLA$_2$ levels (by diaDexus) every 3-6 months as well as CIMT testing (by CardioRisk) every 12-24 months. The Lp-PLA$_2$ should be low-risk and/or decreasing; the CIMT should be stable or preferably decreasing. If not, the problem is: 1) the total LDL-P and/or small LDL-P need to be even lower for this individual patient; 2) the total HDL-P needs to be increased (maybe the measuring cup removing water from the bucket is 'just way too small'); 3) other medical therapies such as ACE-inhibitor, ARB and/or Glitazone/Actos need to be considered; 4) the patient smokes tobacco and/or is being exposed to other such toxins; and/or 5) the patient is 'out-eating' their medications. One way you can prove the latter is with non-fasting advanced lipid testing with the patient doing what they normally do. The advanced lipid test will look somewhat worse, but if it looks way worse, there's something the patient's eating (or drinking) that might be killing them. Since people don't live their lives fasting, it's imperative to determine what's <u>REALLY</u> happening. In such a situation, keep repeating non-fasting TG (or SGGE/VAP/NMR) testing until you identify the problem and then the patient <u>MUST</u> refrain from eating/drinking that particular item in the future.

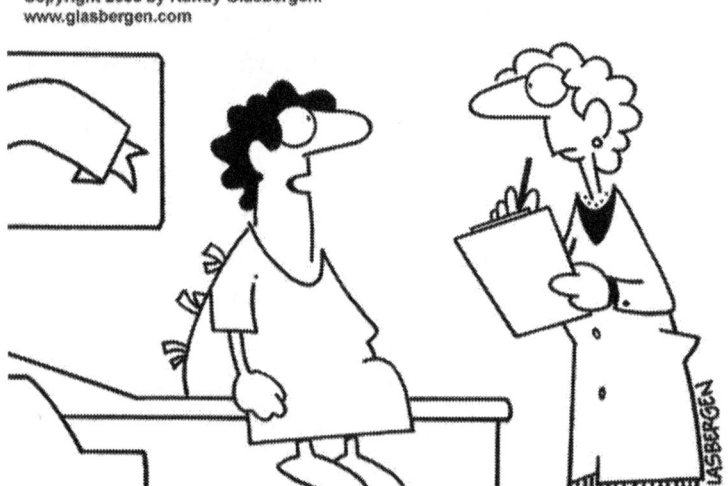

"If I eat all the chocolate I want, I lose my craving for donuts, potato chips, pizza, pie, cookies, pancakes, and pretzels. I think it's a very sensible diet!"

Heart Attack Prevention Institute

Michael P. Varveris, MD—Medical Director
280 N. Tamiami Trail—Naples, FL 34102
(239) 261-3988—FAX (239) 261-1022—www.hapi-naples.com

NIASPAN/ADVICOR—PATIENT INSTRUCTION FORM

- We have decided upon Niaspan/Advicor therapy mainly because multiple large clinical studies with Statins (Crestor, Lescol, Lipitor, Mevacor, Pravachol, Zocor), Fibrates (Lopid, Tricor) and Niacin (Niaspan) used by themselves to treat lipid and/or lipoprotein abnormalities have shown only 20–40% reduction in future heart attacks and strokes on average whereas a few small clinical studies with Statins plus Niacin (such as Advicor) have shown possibly up to 90–95% reduction in future heart attacks and strokes.

- Niaspan/Advicor is to be taken AT BEDTIME (for at least the first week—see below) and as follows:
  - o 1 tablet (500 mg–500/20 mg) at bedtime for 4 weeks then 2 tablets at bedtime
  - o 1 tablet (500 mg–500/20 mg) at bedtime until your next office visit with Dr. Varveris

- <u>You will almost certainly (70% of patients) experience flushing, itching and hot flash symptoms.</u> They usually occur about 1–2 hours after taking the medication and usually last 10–30 minutes. These are NOT HARMFUL, just a nuisance. They are of no negative health consequence. They will decrease in duration and intensity the longer you take the medication (gone within 3 days in 50% of patients and gone within 7 days in 80% of patients). They represent the 'opening' of blood vessels within your body which is one of our major goals. Individuals who experience flushing symptoms must realize that without the Niaspan/Advicor their blood vessels would otherwise thus be 'closed' and 'out-of-shape.' These symptoms are worsened by hot showers, hot beverages, spicy foods, alcohol and taking the medication on an empty stomach. If they are still present and bothersome after one week, you can consider taking the Niaspan/Advicor with breakfast.

- Flushing is decreased by the following:
  - o Take your medication with a meal or low-fat snack (applesauce is a great choice) and consider taking it with a fiber supplement (for the first week or so then stop it)
  - o Take one Aspirin (325 mg) 30 to 60 minutes before Niaspan/Advicor or consider taking 2 Alka-Seltzer tablets containing Aspirin for the first 3 days then one Aspirin as above
  - o Consider taking Benadryl (25–50 mg) at bedtime
  - o If you forget one dose, take your normal dose the next day
  - o If you forget two or more doses in a row, decrease to one tablet per day for one week then resume two tablets per day

♟♟

Chapter Eleven

Final Thoughts from Dr. V

Copyright 2002 by Randy Glasbergen.   www.glasbergen.com

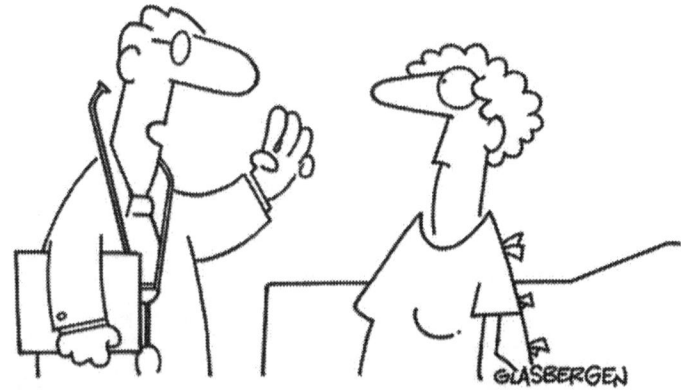

**"In my many years as a doctor, I've found
three things that can help a person lose weight:
shave your head, trim your nails, clean out your navel."**

I must say I had a great time writing the HAPI Heart Diet. I feel like I have raised a wonderful, caring, giving and loving child and am now sending him/her out into the world to help and nurture others. I truly hope you (whether prospective patient or physician) have learned a lot and now look at medical science, health, disease, nutrition, diet, exercise and weight loss in an entirely different light. Remember to enjoy what you do in this regard and I promise you will be successful at it.

If you can take anything away from our experience together, please let it be this: your life and its quality are in your own hands—please recognize that attitude really is everything so think, live and love positively every single day and make your life a great one.

If you want more information or feel the need to contact me personally, you are cordially invited to visit my website: www.hapi-naples.com. TTFN…

Glossary of Medical Abbreviations

AA—arachidonic acid

ABCA1—ATP-binding cassette A1

ACAT—acetyl cholesterol acyltransferase

ACE—angiotensin converting enzyme

ALA—alpha-linolenic acid

Apo—apolipoprotein

ARB—angiotensin II receptor blocker

ARR—absolute risk reduction

ATP—adenosine triphosphate

BAS—bile acid sequestrant

BMR—basal metabolic rate

CAI—cholesterol absorption inhibitor

CCA—common carotid artery

CE—cholesteryl ester

CETP—cholesteryl ester transport protein

CHD—coronary heart disease

CIMT—carotid intima-media thickness

CM-R—chylomicron remnant

CoQ10—coenzyme Q10

CRP—C-reactive protein

CV—cardiovascular

DHA—docosahexaenoic acid

DM—diabetes mellitus

eNOS—endoethelial nitric oxide synthetase

EPA—eicosapentaenoic acid

FBG—fasting blood glucose

FC—free cholesterol

FFA—free fatty acid

GI—glycemic index

HDL—high density lipoprotein

HDL-C—high density lipoprotein cholesterol content

HDL-P—high density lipoprotein particle number/concentration

HL—hepatic lipase

HSL—hormone sensitive lipase

HTN—hypertension

IBW—ideal body weight

IDL—intermediate density lipoprotein

IL—interleukin

IR—insulin resistance

LCAT—lecithin cholesterol acyltransferase

LDL—low density lipoprotein

LDL-C—low density lipoprotein cholesterol content

LDL-P—low density lipoprotein particle number/concentration

LDLr—LDL receptor

LPL—lipoprotein lipase

Lp-PLA$_2$—lipoprotein-associated phospholipase A$_2$

LRP—LDL-related protein

MCP—monocyte chemotactant protein

MS—metabolic syndrome

MUFA—monounsaturated fatty acid

NASH—non alcoholic steatohepatitis

NMR—nuclear magnetic resonance

NNT—number needed to treat

NO—nitric oxide

NPC1L1—Niemann Pick C1 Like 1

PAI—plasminogen activator inhibitor

PL—phospholipid

PPAR—peroxisome proliferator-activated receptor

PUFA—polyunsaturated fatty acid

RDA—recommended daily allowance

RRR—relative risk reduction

SFA—saturated fatty acid

SGGE—segmental gradient gel electrophoresis

SR—scavenger receptor

SREBP—sterol response element binding protein

TC—total cholesterol content

TCM—Traditional Chinese Medicine

TFA—trans fatty acid

TG—triglyceride/triglyceride content

TLC—therapeutic lifestyle changes

TNF—tumor necrosis factor

VAP—vertical auto-profile

VLDL—very low density lipoprotein

VLDL-C—very low density lipoprotein cholesterol

VLDL-P—very low density lipoprotein particle number/concentration

About the Author

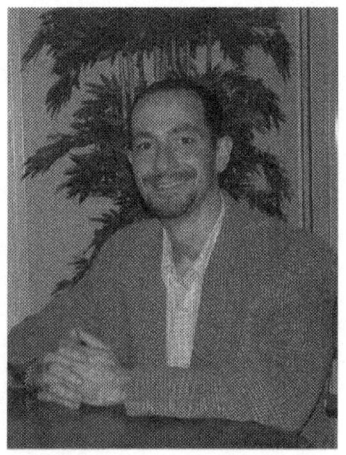

Michael P. Varveris, MD ('Dr. V')

A second generation Greek-American (grandparents coming to the United States through Ellis Island from Smyrna in Asia Minor as well as Kalamata in the Peloponnesus), Dr. V was born in Youngstown, Ohio in 1967. He lived there until graduating high school where he was the Valedictorian of a Boardman High class of about 480 students. He received both his undergraduate degree (BS) as well as medical degree (MD) from the University of Miami in southeast Florida. Invited into Phi Beta Kappa as a junior and inducted into Phi Sigma Phi as a senior, Dr. V was honored as 'Most Outstanding Graduating Senior' in 1989. After medical school, he attended residencies both in Internal Medicine as well as Pathology at Orlando Regional Medical Center in central

Florida where he served as Chief Medical Resident for 18 months and was honored as 'Most Outstanding Resident' in 1997.

Practicing in Naples, Florida since 1997, Dr. V has focused his efforts on preventive cardiology (optimal management of lipoprotein abnormalities, hypertension, type 2 diabetes mellitus and associated behavioral disorders) since 2000 when he opened the Heart Attack Prevention Institute (HAPI). Other than his family, health, exercise, nutrition and cooking/entertaining, Dr. V has interest in Traditional Chinese Medicine (acupuncture and herbal medicine), public speaking, travel, biking, scuba diving, boating, training his three parrots (Frodo, Reagan and Blue Louie) as well as combative martial arts.

978-0-595-38895-0
0-595-38895-7

www.ingramcontent.com/pod-product-compliance
Lightning Source LLC
Chambersburg PA
CBHW030309290526
45785CB00001B/279